# ASHTANGA YOGA

# ASHTANGA YOGA

## The complete mind and body workout

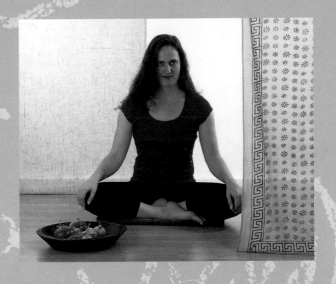

## JULIET PEGRUM

Foreword by
Swami Ambikananda Saraswati

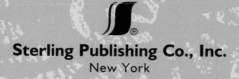

Sterling Publishing Co., Inc.
New York

Library of Congress Cataloging-in-Publication
Data Available

10 9 8 7 6 5 4 3 2 1

Published in 2001 by Sterling Publishing Co., Inc.
387 Park Avenue South, New York, NY 10016

First published in Great Britain in 2001 by
Cico Books Ltd (formerly Cima Books)
32 Great Sutton Street
London EC1V 0NB

Distributed in Canada by Sterling Publishing
C/o Canadian Manda Group
One Atlantic Avenue, Suite 105
Toronto, Ontario, Canada M6K 3E7

Every effort has been made to ensure that all the
information in this book is accurate. However, due
to differing conditions, and individual skills, the
publisher cannot be responsible for any injuries,
losses, and other damages, which may result from
the use of the information in this book.

Printed in Singapore

Sterling ISBN 0-8069-6655-6

## IMPORTANT HEALTH NOTE

Please be aware that the information contained in
this book and the opinions of the author are not a
substitute for medical attention from a qualified
health professional. If you are suffering from any
medical complaint, or are worried about any aspect
of your health, ask your doctor's advice before
proceeding. The publishers can take no responsibility for any injury or illness resulting from the
advice given, or the postures demonstrated within
this volume.

# Contents

# Foreword

by Swami Ambikananda Saraswati

The ancient scriptures tell us that at the dawn of human creation, when the great god Shiva gazed upon the human condition, a great love and sorrow arose in his heart. He saw that humanity had been separated from the state of unconditional perfection that was our heritage to become bound by death, rebirth, and death again, endlessly. Out of this fearsome god's compassion flowed the teaching of Yoga, the promise of freedom.

No matter how deeply we probe it is impossible to discover the origins of yoga. Seals and statues found in excavations of prehistoric sites in India testify that yoga was being practiced millennia before even the appearance of the Vedas. Like all other sacred teachings of its time, it belonged to an oral tradition passed from teacher to disciple. Then around 800 BCE a great sage, Patanjali, who is still revered by Yogis everywhere, codified and wrote down its secrets in pithy aphorisms which became known as the The Eight-limbed Path of Yoga – *Ashtanga yoga.*

Pattabhi Jois has articulated a perspective on Ashtanga yoga that we now, in our age, our cities, and our technologically complex world, can use. Juliet Pegrum, his disciple, holding fast to the teaching of her guru, presents this perspective in a way that makes it accessible to everyone who seeks health and a return to wholeness. Thus, the practice of yoga prescribed in this book offers what Shiva and Patanjali offered – a practice that is a prelude to freedom.

# Ashtanga yoga **mantra**

*Madonna has immortalized the words of the Ashtanga yoga prayer in her popular album* Ray of Light. *Guruji always begins the day with prayers and mantras (sacred words to purify the mind), and this prayer is an important part of yoga practice as it prepares and focuses the mind.*

O M

VANDE GURUNAM CARANARVINDE
SANDARASITA SVATMA SUKHAVA BODHE
NIH SREYASE JANGALIKAYAMANE
SAMSARA HALAHALA MOHASANTYAI

ABAHU PURUSAKARAM
SANKHACAKRASI DHARINAM
SAHASRA SIRASAM SVETAM
PRANAMAMI PATANJALIM

O M

*I pray to the lotus feet of the supreme guru who teaches the*
*Good knowledge, showing the way to knowing the self-awakening*
*Great happiness: who is the doctor of the jungle, able to remove*
*The poison of ignorance of conditioned existence.*

*To Patanjali, an incarnation of Adisesa, white in colour with 1000*
*Radiant heads (in his form as the divine serpent, Ananta), human*
*In form below the shoulders, holding a sword (discrimination), a wheel of*
*Fire (discus of light, representing infinite time),*
*And a conch (divine sound) — to him,*

*I prostrate.*

# How to use this book

*The word Ashtanga in Sanskrit means eight steps or "limbs." There are eight levels in the practice of yoga as formulated by the sage Patanjali in his Yoga Sutras and outlined in this book.*

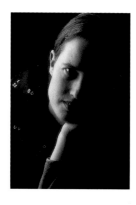

The aspect primarily covered here is step three, the practice of *asana*, which means "steady seat" or "posture." By practicing postures the body becomes stronger, the nervous system is purified, and diseases are removed. Each yoga pose works to realign and detoxify specific organs and muscles (a list of benefits is given beside the poses).

In the Ashtanga system there are six series of poses: the primary series, the intermediate series, and then four advanced series (A, B, C, and D). The series described in this book is the primary or beginners' series. This is known as *yoga chikitsa*, which literally means "yoga therapy" and is specially formulated to rebalance the body and realign the musculoskeletal system.

The primary series consists of approximately 40 poses, which take around an hour and a half to complete. With time, patience, and effort the

## HOW IT WORKS

Orange tabs indicate the two warming-up sequences, known as Salutes to the Sun.

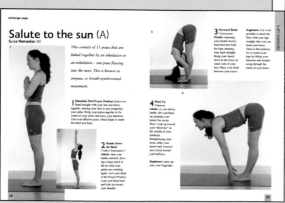

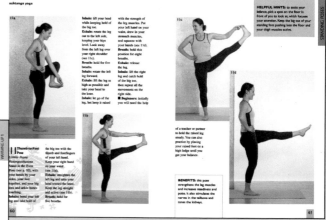

The Standing Pose sequences in Chapter 2 have brown page tabs. Special tips for beginners are included throughout.

entire series can be mastered. Where appropriate, they are presented as sequences of easy and more advanced poses. The poses are given in a precise order, and each one carefully prepares your body for what is to come, so you should not skip or avoid a pose.

Initially you should only go as far in the sequence as your body readily allows; gradually, over time, you will build up the stamina and flexibility that are necessary for the more complex poses. There is no rush to achieve these; yoga is a non-competitive system of self-inquiry. Guru Shri Pattabhi Jois, who is the founder of Ashtanga yoga (see pp. 12–13) says that if you are consistent in your efforts and have respect for your body, then perfection can be attained.

Ashtanga yoga can be practiced by anyone over the age of eight. Women are advised not to practice it during the first two days of menstruation, however, and only until the twelfth week of pregnancy. Women who are more than three months pregnant can still practice particular breathing exercises, which will be of great benefit to them during labor.

If you are new to yoga, then it is always advisable to practice the Ashtanga poses under the guidance of an experienced teacher. Do not try to do the exercises straight from the book. For those of you who are sick, it is recommended that you practice the poses that are beneficial for your particular ailment; this will facilitate you to make a quick recovery. An experienced yoga teacher will be able to guide you in the practice, according to your abilities.

■ No specialist equipment is needed – just a yoga mat.

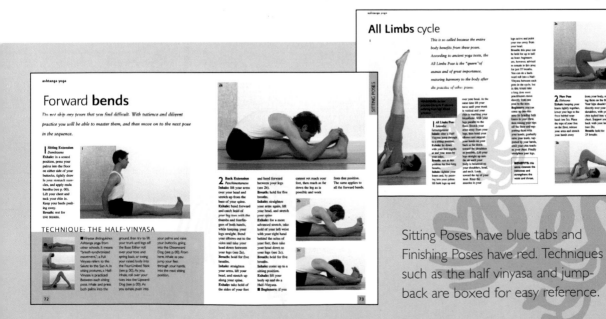

Sitting Poses have blue tabs and Finishing Poses have red. Techniques such as the half vinyasa and jump-back are boxed for easy reference.

# Introduction

The ancient practice of yoga has been traced back to the *Puranas*, Sanskrit chronicles that may date from as early as 6000 B.C. Yoga does not belong to any religion; rather, it is an enduring, profound philosophy that embodies some ideas that are common to all religions. The word *yoga* translates as "the bond," from its root *yuj*, meaning "to yoke" or "harness." This union refers to the highest attainment of the practice, which occurs when the mind becomes fully absorbed in the *atman* or transcendental soul. This ultimate experience is rarely attained. On a day-to-day level, the practice of yoga is a way of life that brings health and harmony to the body, mind, and spirit.

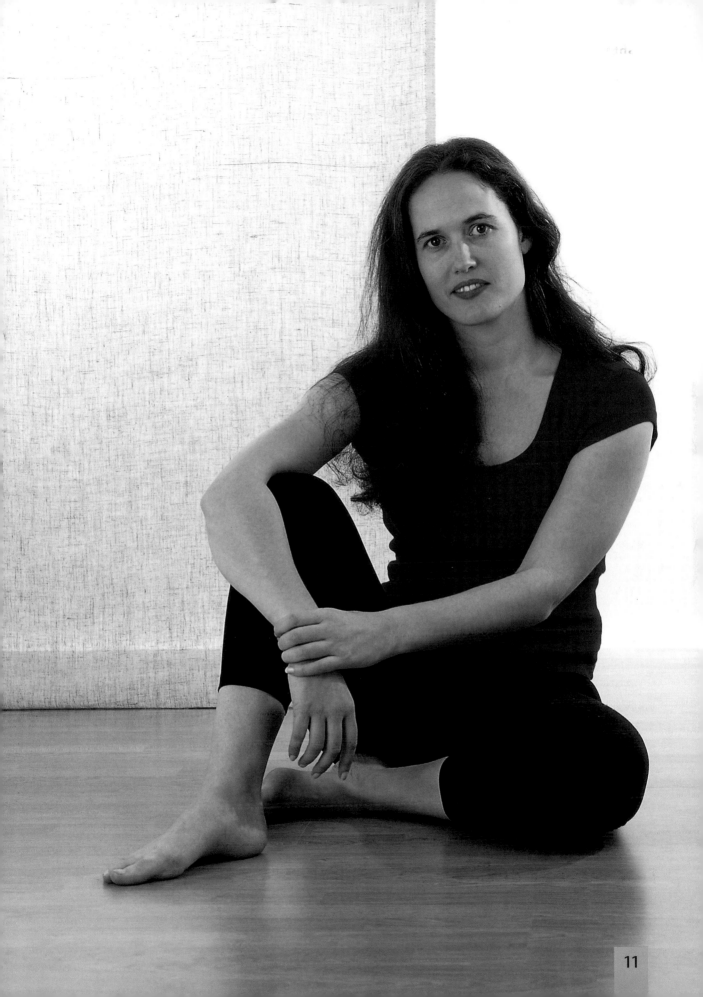

# What is **Ashtanga yoga?**

*Yoga has been passed down from teacher to disciple from ancient times to the present day, and has diversified into many different schools and approaches. The method described in this book is known as Ashtanga yoga.*

Ashtanga yoga is the form taught by Guru Shri Pattabhi Jois (or Guruji, as his students affectionately refer to him), who was born in 1915 in Mysore, in southern India. Guruji has practiced yoga since the age of 12. He was a student of the most famous *yogi* and philosopher of the twentieth century, Krishnamacharya – a great scholar who was solely responsible for inspiring a new wave of interest in yoga within India. While he was researching in Calcutta, Krishnamacharya discovered an ancient text called the *Yoga Korunta*, written on palm leaves by Vamana Rishi, describing an intricate system of linked yoga poses. The word *korunta* can be translated as "the master yoga" or "king of yogis." This text is thought to be more than 2,000 years old. Krishnamacharya recited the *slokas,* or verses, to Guru Shri Pattabhi Jois, who faithfully recorded them and collated the series that became known as Ashtanga yoga.

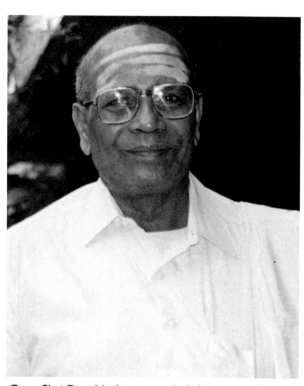

Guru Shri Pattabhi Jois recorded the series of poses from the *Yoga Korunta,* the basis of Ashtanga.

Guruji still teaches from his family home. There is a small, windowless room at the rear at the house, which can barely accommodate 12 students at a time, mat-to-mat. The confined space is ideal for the generation of intense heat, which is an essential part of Ashtanga yoga practice. The atmosphere in the tiny room is highly charged and concentrated, filled with the sibilant sound of the practitioner's *ujjayi* breathing.

# Working with **a guru**

*A guru is a vital component of the Ashtanga yoga system, passing on the wealth of his accumulated spiritual wisdom to his disciples. It is vital that the Ashtanga poses are passed on accurately to a student.*

It is said that if you are filled with a longing for the truth, a *guru* (teacher or leader) will appear. *Gu* can be translated as darkness, heaviness, or responsibility; *ru* is the opposite, meaning lightness. The guru is therefore responsible for leading us from darkness or ignorance toward the ultimate transcendental knowledge or light. The guru-disciple relationship forms an intrinsic part of Indian culture. Sacred knowledge was traditionally passed on verbally, so that the blessings of the lineage would be transferred in an unbroken chain – this is known as *shakti-pata*, or direct spiritual transmission. The bond between a teacher and a disciple is so strong that it is believed to transverse lifetimes. Because a guru is a person who has reached enlightenment, or *samadhi* (the ultimate experience of yoga), through the grace of his own teacher, he is able to initiate you by means of an unbroken chain of master-disciple initiation.

Though the guru-disciple relationship functions very well in the East, it is often misunderstood and even abused in the West. I would suggest that you avoid self-styled Western gurus and look instead for a knowledgeable, experienced yoga teacher who can pass on the poses correctly.

# Yoga philosophy:
## the eight limbs

Ashtanga refers to the famous eight "limbs" of yoga that are the subject of the *Yoga Sutras* (or sayings) written by Patanjali between 400 and 200 B.C. Patanjali is known as the architect of yoga because he compiled and systematized the existing knowledge of yoga, giving it a philosophical shape. It is essential to have a basic understanding of Patanjali's *Yoga Sutras* to bring the mind and sense organs under control, for the achievement of enlightenment.

The aim of yoga is to control mental activity. One of Guruji's famous answers, when asked a question about yoga, is "Do your practice and all is coming" – meaning that to grasp something intellectually is not comparable to the experiential knowledge of a subject. Overstimulating the intellect in an effort to understand yoga is counter-productive. The classic example is trying to imagine what sugar tastes like if you have never eaten it. However, as a beginner it is important to have some intellectual understanding in order to propel you deeper into the path of yoga. As Krishnamacharya said, "Learn the scriptures and, only when you know them, discard them completely."

**THE PATANJALI** *YOGA SUTRA*

"Let one bring *chitta* [mind] under control by withdrawing it, wherever it wanders away, drawn by the various objects of sight."

The aim of yoga is union with the inner self, the essence of all things. Patanjali says that only when the mind is completely still, without disturbance, can the true nature of self be experienced.

When the mind is quiet, there is no duality of subject and object – it is free to rest in its own intrinsic qualities, which are joy, equanimity, bliss, and compassion. This may appear to be a simple task, but in my experience, when trying to remain still for just 20 minutes to meditate, the mind conjures up an array of distractions.

Guruji likens the untamed mind to a monkey being led by the five senses, jumping from one thought to the next, completely absorbed in the external world, inquisitive, and restless. The wisdom of yoga says that only by turning your attention within will you find true, lasting peace and contentment.

"**YOGA IS FREEDOM** FROM MENTAL DISTURBANCE."

## THE OUTER PRACTICES

The yamas (which translate as "forbearance") are the first step and consist of five abstentions. The yamas establish an ethical code of conduct, and are a means to regain balance in your life. The abstentions include non-harming, truthfulness, non-stealing, non-sensuality, and non-possessiveness. They are referred to as "the great vows" and they continue throughout all levels of yoga practice. There is never a point at which you can say, "Now I am a great yogi and beyond the force of my actions." The yamas help to regulate the disturbances of body and mind created by desires.

### STEP ONE: *THE YAMAS (OR RESTRAINTS – YOUR ATTITUDE TOWARD OTHERS)*

"Freeing himself from individuality, force, pride, desire, anger, and acquisitiveness, unpossessive, tranquil, he is at one with the infinite spirit."

### a. Non-harming *(ahimsa)*

On an extreme level, this translates as "not killing"; on a more subtle level, it incorporates angry thoughts and a willingness to harm any sentient life – and that includes yourself.

# THE EIGHT LIMBS

Patanjali's eight "limbs" highlight the path by which disturbances (which distract the mind from the experience of yoga) can be removed. The first four steps consist of the outer practices:

**1** restraints *(yama)*
**2** observances *(niyama)*
**3** postures *(asana)*
**4** breath control *(pranayama)*.

The second four steps consist of the inner practices:

**5** sense withdrawal *(pratyahara)*
**6** concentration *(dharana)*
**7** meditation *(dhyana)*
**8** self-realization *(samadhi)*, when the eternal self alone shines in the mind.

The last four are collectively referred to as Raja yoga, or mind control.

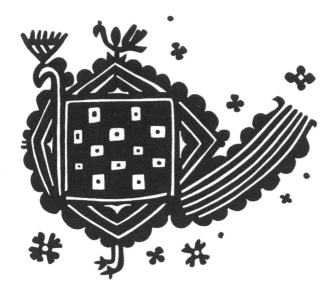

### b. Truthfulness *(staya)*

If someone is aligned in thought, word, and deed, then the mind is at ease. Any deception, in the hope of winning some sort of advantage over another person or situation, should be avoided.

### c. Non-stealing *(asteya)*

This means not taking or using things that belong to others, without their consent.

### d. Non-sensuality *(brahmacharya)*

This implies moderation of the senses, including any excess or debauchery in food, sex, or drugs. Managing the senses promotes health, reduces heightened mental activity, and produces more vital energy.

### e. Non-possessiveness *(aparigraha)*

This means avoiding the overwhelming desire to have what others possess – whether this be material objects or personal characteristics. Non-possessiveness leads to inner freedom and contentment in life.

By withdrawing from external objects, you begin the process of training your mind, harnessing your energy, and bringing your awareness back to yourself. Other than to sustain bodily functions, external objects will not provide true happiness, peace, and contentment. Yoga is the art of life management, leading to the discovery of joy and purpose within yourself. Many people believe that life would be devoid of pleasure without the support of external stimuli. In reality, objects that appear pleasurable (such as rich food) can lead to all manner of painful physical and emotional problems. Buddhist philosophy likens sensual pleasures to honey on a razor blade – they appear to be sweet, but have painful consequences. In fact, the less you are driven by external objects, the more you are at liberty to appreciate and enjoy them.

## STEP TWO: *THE NIYAMAS (OR OBSERVANCES – YOUR ATTITUDE TOWARD YOURSELF)*

The niyamas, or devotions, develop as a direct consequence of the five yama abstentions. They refocus the mind on the inner quest for fulfilment, rather than on dependence upon external circumstances.

### a. Purity *(saucha)*

The term purity means both cleansing and the proper nourishment of the body and the mind. External cleanliness includes your living environment as well as your personal bodily cleanliness. Internal cleanliness incorporates both the foods that you eat and mental cleanliness. Negative thoughts or malevolent feelings toward others should always be avoided.

### b. Contentment *(santosha)*

This implies complete acceptance of life's circumstances at any given moment.

### c. Self-discipline (tapas)

This means putting effort into your spiritual practice, which will lead to self-mastery.

### d. Self-study (svahyaya)

This is the study of "the self" (not oneself), by reading the scriptures and the lives of the saints.

### e. Self-surrender (ishvara pranidhana)

Self-surrender means dedication to the idea of supreme selfhood, which involves the surrender of your whole self to the concept of liberation.

## STEP THREE: THE ASANAS (OR POSTURES)

"Being the first accessory of Hatha yoga, asana...should be practiced to gain steady posture, health, and lightness of body." *Hatha Yoga Pradipika*, ch. 1, v. 19

Asana practice is generally referred to as Hatha yoga, meaning forceful or physical yoga, and forms the third "limb." The word asana literally translates as "seat," or steady posture. Through asana practice, the subtle energy channels known as *nadis* (which run throughout the body) are purified, conditioning the body to enable it to maintain a steady posture in which to meditate. Yoga philosophy regards the body as the temple of the divine spirit and therefore it should be cared for and appreciated as a divine gift.

The poses are much more than physical exercises; they are a holistic practice that works on many different levels. They tone the internal organs, regulate the hormones, strengthen the nervous system, build a strong and flexible muscular physique, and produce mental equilibrium.

Through the practice of asana, awareness, concentration, and meditation are cultivated – these being the final steps in the development of yoga.

There are said to be 840,000 different poses, first described by Shiva, a popular Hindu deity referred to in the *Puranas* as the founder of yoga. There are supposedly as many poses as there are species of animal living in the universe – and many of them are named after animals and vegetation. Yoga is a celebration of life, realizing the divine spark within all creation.

Asana practice is the aspect of the whole yoga system that has attracted greatest attention in the West. Its purpose, however, is to prepare the body for self-realization, or the ultimate experience of yoga: samadhi. Asana yoga is referred to in the *Gheranda Samhita* (an ancient text on yoga) as training in hardiness, which is the first rung on the ladder that leads to the royal heights of Raja yoga, or mind control.

The mind-body relationship is extremely subtle, and Hatha yoga is the area in which to explore and observe this interaction. The practice requires presence of mind from moment to moment in order to overcome fear and limiting belief patterns. Eventually, the body and mind will move together in harmony, being absorbed into the eternal.

## STEP FOUR: *PRANAYAMA* (OR BREATH CONTROL)

"By whom the breathing has been controlled, by him the activities of the mind have also been controlled." *Hatha Yoga Pradipika*, ch. 4, v. 21

The next "limb" is pranayama. *Prana* translates as "life force," being a subtle energy that is said to pervade all phenomena and is present in breath, along with the gross element of air. *Ayama* means "expansion," and so the word pranayama signifies the "expansion of the life force." Breath control has three phases, known as inhalation *(puraka)*, retention *(kumbhaka)*, and exhalation *(rechaka)* – and is the gateway to unlocking deeper aspects of the self, as breathing is an unconscious reflex of the body. As stated in the *Hatha Yoga Pradipika:*
"Mind is the master of the senses and breathing is the master of the mind."

The strong connection between breathing and the sympathetic nervous system can be observed by noticing how shallow your breathing becomes when you are afraid or anxious. By deepening your breathing, you calm the mind, increasing the oxygen supply to the body's physiological system, which is vital for optimum health. There are, however, different varieties of breath-control techniques; pranayama is usually taught only after a degree of proficiency in Hatha yoga has been established.

Patanjali emphasizes relaxed breathing. There should be no external restrictions (such as the wearing of tight clothing) and no internal restrictions (such as anxiety, or any undue forcing or holding of the breath). He says that when breath-ing is free and relaxed, a veil that obscures the goal of enlightenment fades away and the mind becomes ready for fixed attentiveness.

You should not practice breath control without the guidance of an experienced teacher, or you could disrupt the subtle energies of the body. However, if pranayama is practiced properly it has great therapeutic value, especially for breath-related problems such as asthma and coughs, and more generally it invigorates the entire system.

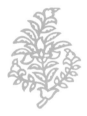

The next four "limbs" – pratyahara, dharana, dhyana, and samadhi – pertain to the states that are experienced in deep meditation. It is important to seek a qualified meditation instructor to guide you through this practice, once your body and mind have reached a steady, balanced level through practice of the first four steps. As the *Hatha Yoga Pradipika* (ch. 2, v. 76) states: "No success in Raja Yoga, without Hatha Yoga, and no success in Hatha Yoga without Raja Yoga. One should, therefore, practice both of these until complete success is gained."

## STEP FIVE: *PRATYAHARA* (OR SENSE WITHDRAWAL)

"The mysteries are to be understood by the heart and not the mind."

Breath control is the path between the outer and inner worlds and begins the transition from the four outer stages of yoga practice to the four inner stages. The fifth "limb" is termed "the retraction of the senses"; it is the withdrawal of the mind from attention to sensuous appearances, which in turn leads directly to the sixth step. The first five steps of the yoga disciplines are collectively known as *sadhana*, or the method of self-realization.

## STEP SIX: DHARANA (OR CONCENTRATION)

"Mind and understanding fixed on me, free from doubt, you will come to me."

The sixth "limb" is known as concentration, or fixed attention, and is an extension of the previous step – holding the mind steady on a single point and not being diverted by seductive sounds, smells, tactile impulses, or distracting thoughts. Thoughts will continuously arise, but by concentrating on a fixed point or object, such as your breathing, you will gain the ability to observe your thoughts without becoming involved in them. After some time, the mind begins to settle, a degree of equanimity starts to develop, and you are no longer disturbed by its various activities. By focusing your attention, you are led naturally to the seventh stage.

## STEP SEVEN: DHYANA (OR MEDITATION)

"When his thought ceases, checked by exercise of discipline, he is content with the self, seeing the self through himself."

The seventh "limb", dhyana, involves the deepening of concentration. Commonly translated as "meditation," dhyana is a further unification of

consciousness, at which point discursive thoughts and creative imagination begin to subside. This leads directly to the final stage.

## STEP EIGHT: SAMADHI (OR SELF-REALIZATION)

"Whoever knows me without delusion as the supreme spirit of man knows all there is."

The "self" referred to in this instance does not mean your ego-related or small self, but rather the essence that is left once all associations and impressions of a distinct inherent self have been removed – simple, pure awareness. Consciousness in its pure state is likened to a flawless diamond, because it is indestructible. Diamonds are by far the hardest substance known to humankind and, like pure awareness, a perfect diamond is completely transparent and invisible.

The eighth "limb" is known as samadhi, or ecstasy, whereby the mind becomes as unconscious of itself as it is of any other object. When the life force (*prana*) is compressed into the spinal column (*sushumna nadi*) through the practice of yoga, the mind becomes completely absorbed in the soul. Then the body resonates with the divine, which is a state of pure bliss.

There are believed to be different levels of samadhi, although the ultimate experience of it is very rarely attained. The *Hatha Yoga Pradipika* (ch. 4, v. 9) states: "Indifference to worldly enjoyment is very difficult to obtain, and equally difficult to obtain is the knowledge of the realities. It is very hard to achieve the condition of samadhi, without the favor of a true guru."

# How to **practice**

*"When the body becomes lean, the face glows with delight, anahatanada [kundalini] manifests and the eyes are clear, the body is healthy, bindu under control and the appetite increases, then one should know that the nadis are purified and success in yoga is approaching."* Hatha Yoga Pradipika, ch. 2, v. 78

Ashtanga yoga is a dynamic form of yoga that synchronizes the movements, the breathing, and the "locks" (*bandhas*), which in turn focus the mind. The poses occur in a particular fluid sequence, each linked together by the breath. This is known as *vinyasa*, which translates as "breath-synchronized movement." It is the use of vinyasa that separates Ashtanga yoga from other forms. As Vamana Rishi states in the *Yoga Korunta*, "O yogi, don't do asana without vinyasa." Because of its dynamic form, Ashtanga yoga has incorrectly been referred to as "power yoga." Do not be put off by this. With patience and consistent effort, even the more difficult poses can be mastered. You will quickly build strength and stamina using the vinyasa system, while the heat that is generated through the practice promotes increased flexibility.

The advantages of the poses are many: the body becomes strong, the organs are toned, the mind becomes steady and focused, and longevity is increased. It is not possible to pursue a spiritual life if the body is not strong.

## PRACTICAL POINTS

### ■ TIME
The best times to practice are in the early morning at sunrise, or in the early evening at sunset. The benefit of practicing in the morning before the day starts is that the mind is clear and alert, though the body is generally stiff; whereas in the evening the body is looser, but the mind is overactive or dull.

### ■ PLACE
The surroundings should be pleasant and inspiring. It is best to practice in a dust-free room, which is clear of clutter and distractions. The room needs to be well heated, with no drafts. The asana can also be practiced outdoors if the weather is warm and not too windy. Sandy beaches are beautiful settings, but can be problematic for asana practice and are more suited to meditation.

### ■ PREPARATION
The poses are best performed on an empty stomach, so it is advisable not to eat anything for at least three hours beforehand. That is one advantage of practicing first thing in the morning. Ideally the bowels should also be emptied before practice.

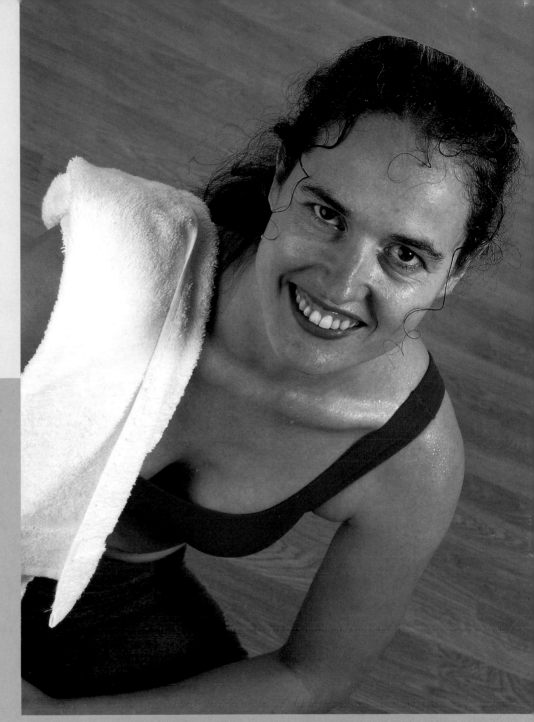

Ashtanga yoga produces copious perspiration, but the essential minerals and salts should be rubbed back into the body.

## ■ TIMES TO AVOID

Do not practice on the days of the new and full moon. Women should not practice during the first two days of menstruation (and especially not inverted poses) or after the 12th week of pregnancy (except for certain breathing exercises).

## ■ CLOTHING

Wear loose or stretchy clothing that does not restrict the circulation.

## ■ EQUIPMENT

To avoid possible injury, use a non-slip mat that is specifically designed for yoga.

## ■ BREATHING

Breathe only through the nose and keep your mouth closed. Even, regular breathing should be maintained throughout your yoga practice. Often, in difficult poses, there is a tendency to hold the breath.

# Breath **control**

*Pranayama, or breath control, helps to stabilize the mind, since the body and mind are inseparably linked. Mental stress is thought to cause numerous ailments, from weight loss to heart problems, but when the mind is steady and tranquil, this helps the body to remain healthy. The system of breath control known as ujjayi breathing is an integral part of the physical practice of the Ashtanga system, along with the gaze (drishti), meditation (dhyana), and the internal locks, known as the bandhas: mula bandha and uddiyana bandha.*

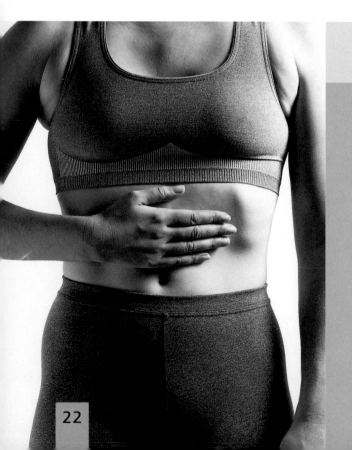

## UJJAYI BREATHING

■ Ujjayi breathing is one of the most important aspects of Ashtanga; it is said to be the thread from which the poses hang. Each movement is performed on an exhalation *(rechaka)* or an inhalation *(puraka)*. The breath should be drawn in and released only through the nose. By contracting the muscles at the base of the throat and narrowing the epiglottis, you create a soft snoring sound at the back of the throat. This technique helps regulate the flow of breath, bringing awareness to your breathing. With more difficult poses, your breathing will become faster and more shallow, and at this point you consciously begin to deepen and calm it, which in turn calms the mind.

## UJJAYI BREATHING (VICTORIOUS BREATH)

"Respiration being disturbed, the mind becomes disturbed. By restraining respiration, the yogi gets steadiness of mind." *Hatha Yoga Pradipika,* ch. 2, v. 2

The form of breathing taught by Guruji in conjunction with the movements is called ujjayi breathing, translated as "victorious breath." This is explained in the *Hatha Yoga Pradipika* (ch. 2, v. 51) as follows: "Having closed the opening of the *nadi* [larynx], the air should be drawn up in such a way that it goes touching from the throat to the chest, and making a noise while passing."

The breath is said to be a combination of the gross element of air and the subtle life force known as prana, which is omnipresent throughout the cosmos. Prana is believed to flow throughout the subtle body by means of the system of channels called nadis (of which there are at least 72,000 in the body). Through breath control, or pranayama, the yogi clears the nadis of obstructions and is able to control the flow of prana. Increased prana leads to increased awareness and vitality. As the *Hatha Yoga Pradipika* (ch. 2, v. 5) states: "When the whole system of nadis, which is full of impurities, is cleaned, then the yogi becomes able to control prana."

## DRISHTI (GAZE)

"When the yogi remains inwardly attentive to the Brahman, keeping the mind and the prana absorbed and the sight steady, as if seeing everything, while in reality seeing nothing outside, above, or below…" *Hatha Yoga Pradipika*, ch. 4, v. 36

Holding the mind steady by fixing your gaze on a single point, and not being distracted by seductive sounds, smells, tactile impulses, or stray thoughts, comprises part of the sixth "limb" and is incorporated into the Ashtanga system through the dristi, or steady gaze. Intrinsic to each pose is a particular focal point – for example, the navel, tip of the nose, or midpoint between the eyebrows. Keeping your gaze fixed on a certain spot is another device for steadying the mind. During your practice, you will notice that wandering eyes are accompanied by distracting thoughts. Traditionally, yoga was practiced in solitude, not in groups, and for good reason. In a yoga class with 20 or more students, there are myriad distractions (such as comparing yourself to others, and wondering who has just entered the room). However, you will soon discover that, no matter where you are, thoughts continuously arise. By concentrating on your

■ By using the ujjayi technique, and without exerting too much control, your breathing will automatically deepen and your diaphragm will widen. The expansion of the diaphragm presses on certain internal organs, such as the liver and stomach, and gently stimulates and massages them. Acting like a set of bellows, ujjayi breathing also activates the internal fire *(agni)*, which generates digestive and psychosomatic heat that purifies the inner channels (nadis). The intense heat that is produced enables the body to be far more pliable and flexible than normal, and usually difficult poses become easier to accomplish.

breathing and keeping your gaze fixed, you gain the ability to observe thoughts without being involved and distracted. In time, the mind begins to settle down and a degree of equanimity develops, for you are no longer tossed around by your own emotional response to situations.

The four drishti points used in Ashtanga are the nose, thumb, navel, and "third eye" (located in the middle of the forehead, between the eyebrows).

## DHYANA (MEDITATION)

"One should become void in and void out, and void like a pot in the space. Full inside and full outside, like a jar in the ocean." *Hatha Yoga Pradipika,* ch. 4, v. 55

Once the Ashtanga series is practiced with ease, your breathing becomes even, and your gaze is steady, the active mind begins to become absorbed and pure awareness increases. At this point the fluid series of movements becomes a moving meditation, and a state of contemplation has been reached. This is dhyana, which forms the seventh "limb" of Ashtanga practice.

The mind is now alert and active, aware of each subtle movement of the body, yet relaxed. The mind becomes perfectly sustained in the present moment, and an indescribable feeling of joy and elation is experienced in the body. According to the *Yoga Darshana* (ch. 3, v. 2): "To keep the mind solely on one subject is contemplation."

## BANDHAS (INTERNAL LOCKS)

"The person who desires to cross the ocean of existence, let him go to a retired place and practice in secrecy this *mudra* [hand position]. By the practice of it, the *vayu* [prana] is undoubtedly controlled." *Gheranda Samhita*, ch. 3, v. 16–17

The bandhas, or internal locks, are muscular contractions that aid yoga practice. The two internal locks that are essential to the successful practice of Ashtanga yoga are known as mula bandha and uddiyana bandha. By contracting certain muscle groups, you affect the physical, pranic, and psychic bodies. Through the force of the internal locks you awaken dormant cosmic energy (*kundalini*), which is the vehicle for the expansion of consciousness. As this rises and begins its journey up the spinal-column nadi, it pierces the psychic knots (*granthis*) located in each energy centre (*chakra*).

Traditionally the bandhas were taught in secret, and only after a student had mastered many

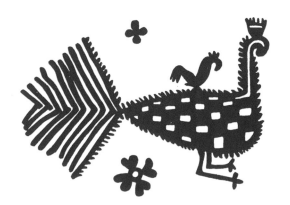
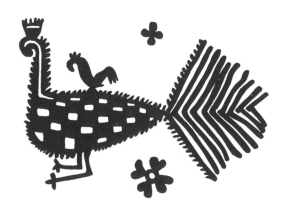

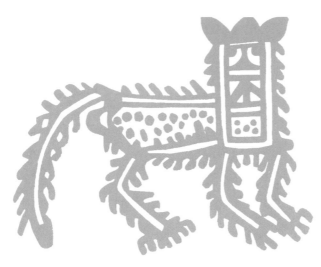

complex asanas. As a beginner, it is most important to familiarize yourself with the poses; only when you are comfortable with them should you turn your attention to the internal locks.

## MULA BANDHA (ROOT LOCK)

"Even an old man becomes young by constantly practicing mula bandha." *Hatha Yoga Pradipika,* ch. 3, v. 64

*Mula* means root and *bandha* means lock, and mula bandha is believed to be the most important of the internal locks, whereby the area between the anus and the scrotum or clitoris is contracted. Mula bandha therefore involves the contraction of the perineal muscle group, which stimulates the parasympathetic fibers that emerge from the base of the spinal column. This promotes a deep sense of relaxation and wellbeing.

The perineum is connected to two groups of muscles common to both sexes: those of the anal region (which are larger) and those of the genital region (which are smaller). Both areas are interrelated. This group of muscles usually only functions during urination, defecation, and orgasm – all of which are subconscious or autonomic activities – and gaining conscious control of them is difficult and takes a degree of practice.

Mula bandha also has pranic and psychic ramifications. The concentration required to sustain awareness of the lock sharpens the mind. Over time, with persistence and practice, your mental energy is refined and becomes a potent force of ever-increasing awareness and bliss.

## UDDIYANA BANDHA (FLYING CONTRACTION)

"Uddiyana is so called because the great bird prana, tied to it, flies without being fatigued." *Hatha Yoga Pradipika*, ch. 3, v. 55

Drawing in the navel performs uddiyana bandha, which literally means "to fly up," so that the abdominal muscles move toward the back. This technique massages the internal organs, adrenal organs, digestive tract, kidneys, and solar plexus, and gives support and expansion to the lungs. The lower spine is protected, by keeping the stomach contracted during asana practice. By squeezing the solar plexus, a flood of energy is released into the abdomen and chest. Uddiyana bandha conditions the sympathetic nervous system, helping to remove the effects of stress.

These three ingredients – ujjayi breathing, mula bandha, and uddiyana bandha – should be kept in mind throughout your practice. Generally, mula bandha and uddiyana bandha are applied in every posture, unless otherwise stated, but there are certain poses in which the locks should be released, and these are indicated later in the book. By harmonizing the poses with your breathing, and by practicing the two internal locks, you produce an intense heat that helps to make the body flexible.

# Nadis: energy channels

*"The vayu [prana] does not enter the nadis so long as they are full of impurities."* Gheranda Samhita, ch. 5, v. 35

There is a vast network of subtle energy channels, known as nadis (meaning "flow"), that crisscross the entire body. When this intricate network is cleansed, energy flows freely throughout the system. Yoga texts differ on the exact number of nadis, but there are at least 72,000, of which three are of primary importance. These are the *pingala nadi*, the *ida nadi*, and the *sushumna nadi*, which form the prime conduits of energy throughout the system. One of the nadis (the pingala) is positive, one (the ida) is negative, and the other (the sushumna) is neutral – just as in any electrical circuit.

Hatha yoga is one of the most important steps in obtaining enlightenment, or samadhi, which is achieved by purification of the nadis through yoga poses. The word Hatha comes from *ha*, meaning "sun," which represents the pingala (positive) nadi. This is situated to the right of the sushumna nadi (central channel or spinal column), and according to most yogic scriptures it terminates in the right nostril. It is associated with the physical faculties of the body and is the masculine energy. *Tha*, on the other hand, means "moon" and refers to the ida (negative) nadi. This is situated to the left of the sushumna nadi. It is generally believed to commence at the base of the spine and extend to the left nostril, coiling around the central channel. It is associated with mental faculties and is the female energy. Both the ida

and the pingala nadis emerge from the muladhara-chakra (see p. 28) and cross the central channel at four of the energy centers (chakras); they join at the ajna-chakra, the sixth energy point. The sushumna nadi is said to flow from the base of the spine along the spinal column to the crown of the head. When it is activated, both your mental and physical faculties become balanced and the mind is calm. This unification of energy is brought about by the practice of Hatha yoga.

The yoga texts describe how, through the practice of asana, cosmic energy (kundalini, often represented in Indian iconography as a coiled serpent) is said to rise along the sushumna nadi. This energy supposedly lies dormant at the base of the spine in the *khanda* (foundation or base) just above the muladhara-chakra. The khanda is the area of the body where the three primary nadis meet and where all 72,000 nadis originate. It corresponds to the "horsetail" in the physical body – the nerve bundle that emerges from the base of the spinal column. As cosmic energy rises upward along the sushumna nadi it pierces the psychic knots or blockages, as a result of which a mortal may become immortal. It has been compared to "the piercing of a bamboo by means of a heated iron rod."

# HOW TO DRINK

■ "The perspiration exuding from the exertion of practice should be rubbed into the body (and not wiped), as by doing so the body becomes strong."

*Hatha Yoga Pradipika*, ch. 11, v. 13

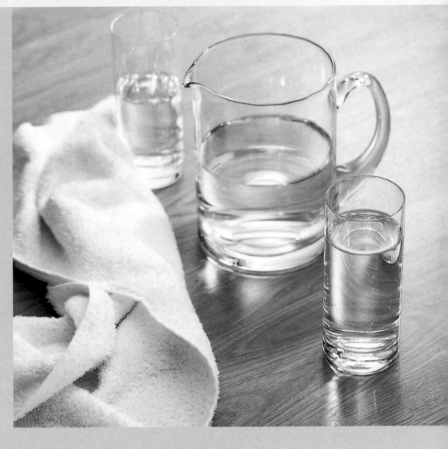

■ The intense heat that builds in the body from the combination of movement, internal locks, and breathing produces profuse perspiration. Sweating removes toxins from the body, but it also releases essential salts and minerals, and it is therefore advisable to rub the moisture back into your body after practice, so that the minerals can be reabsorbed. The advice given by Guruji is to avoid exposing your body to the open air in an attempt to dry the sweat, as this will cause a sapping of your vital energies and will create weakness in the body. He recommends waiting for at least one and a half hours after practice before venturing out into the open air, and half an hour before taking a hot bath, to give your body time to reabsorb the essential salts and minerals.

■ Because of the excess fluid that is lost from the body during practice, it is important to replenish the system with fresh water, but it is not recommended that you drink either before or during your workout. It is best to wait for 20 minutes after the workout, by which time your body will have cooled down. Do not drink ice-cold water, which is too shocking for the system, but choose fresh mineral water at room temperature. If you are feeling particularly dehydrated, it is good occasionally to mix a sachet of rehydration formula into the water (this can be purchased over the counter at a good pharmacy). Another fast method for rejuvenating the system is to drink freshly squeezed fruit or vegetable juices, which are also full of vital nutrients.

# Chakras: energy wheels

*"This she-serpent [kundalini] should be awakened by catching hold of her tail. By the force of Hatha, the sakti [kundalini energy] leaves her sleep, and starts upward."* Hatha Yoga Prādipika, ch. 3, v. 5

Yoga philosophy describes an inner or psychic dimension to the body, often referred to as the "subtle body," which is not visible to the physical eye. The subtle body is crisscrossed by the network of nadis along which the energy of prana flows. Chakras translate as "wheels," and are energy centers situated along the subtle body. Most yoga schools identify seven major such vortices, located along the central sushumna nadi. It is believed that each of these centers corresponds to higher levels of consciousness. Normally certain levels are blocked to the ordinary person by psychic knots (granthis), of which there are thought to be three; they block the energy current from flowing along the central channel. However, through yoga, the dormant cosmic energy at the base of the spine is awakened and rises along the sushumna nadi, piercing the knots as it goes, and thereby consciousness is expanded. As the *Hatha Yoga Pradipika* (ch. 4, v. 71–2) states: "The airs are united into one and begin moving in the middle channel... By this means the Vishnu knot [in the throat] is pierced, which is indicated by the highest pleasure experienced."

The seven chakras are:

### 1. Muladhara-chakra
This is located at the base of the body, at the perineum (the region between the anus and the genitals). This chakra is stimulated by the action of the root lock, or mula bandha. This is the location of cosmic energy and the source of the sushumna nadi.

### 2. Svadhishthana-chakra
This chakra is situated in the genital area.

### 3. Manipura-chakra
This psychoenergetic center is located at the level of the navel. It is the site of the triangular region of fire, the fiery digestive energy center.

### 4. Anahata-chakra
This is located at the heart center, believed to be the seat of the divine. It is the site of the first of the psychic knots, the Brahma granthi.

### 5. Vishuddha-chakra
This chakra at the throat is the location of the second psychic knot, the Vishnu granthi.

### 6. Ajna-chakra
This is situated in the center of the head, between the eyebrows, and is also known as the "third eye." It is the location of the final psychic knot, the Rudra granthi, the piercing of which is said to produce all kinds of psychic powers.

### 7. Sahasrara-chakra
This chakra is located at the crown of the head and is known as the "thousand-petaled lotus." It is the final destination of cosmic energy.

# HOW TO EAT

■ "He who practices Yoga without moderation of diet incurs various diseases and obtains no success."

*Gheranda Samhita*, ch. 5, v. 16

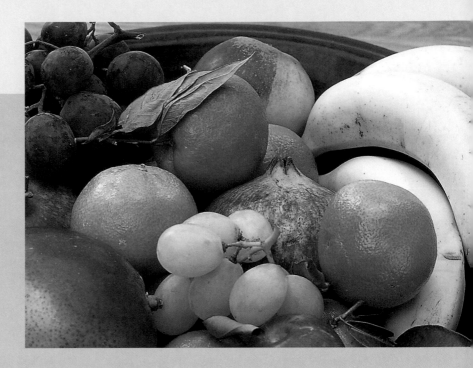

Food is one of the main human preoccupations and has a powerful effect on our mind and emotions. According to the scriptures pertaining to yoga, the consumption of foods either enhances or hinders the practice of yoga.

In India, it is believed that foods are a combination of particular energies. There are three energies, known as *sattva, rajas,* and *tamas,* of which all manifest objects are comprised in different proportions. The three energies and how they affect the body are covered in great depth in the system of Ayurveda, which literally translates as "life science."

Sattva is a clear, lucid energy and can be felt internally as periods of joy, clarity, and efficiency. Tamas is the polar opposite – its energy is heavy and inert, and it can be experienced as moments of laziness and lethargy. The third energy, rajas, is caused by the tension created in the opposition of sattva and tamas. Rajas energy is restless and active, and it can be experienced as manic energy. It drives us to a state of either lethargy or clarity.

## Good foods for yoga

The best foods for yoga are those that enhance sattva energy (such as rice, yogurt, legumes, ginger, milk, and sugar), as they create a more tranquil state of mind. Foods containing tamas energy (such as red meat or rich, stodgy food) – and overeating – produce apathy. Foods containing rajas energy (such as hot and spicy foods) affect the mind and heat the body, causing restlessness. Most yoga practitioners favor a vegetarian diet.

■ "Bitter, sour, saltish, hot, green vegetables, fermented, oily, mixed with til [sesame] seed, rape seed, intoxicating liquors, fish, meat, curds, chhaasa pulses [chick peas], plums, oil cake, asafetida, garlic, onion, etc., should not be eaten." *Hatha Yoga Pradipika*, ch. 1, v. 61

■ "Wheat, rice, barley, shastik [a kind of rice], good corns, milk, ghee, sugar, butter, sugar candy, honey, dried ginger, parwal [a vegetable], the five vegetables, moong [mung beans], pure water, these are very beneficial to those who practice yoga." *Hatha Yoga Pradipika*, ch. 1, v. 64

# How to **relax**

*Letting go of the tension in every muscle is an integral part of yoga.*

*Due to poor postural habits, excessive strain is placed on various muscle groups, which causes pain. Relaxation and pain relief may be elusive, even during sleep. All too often we turn to the quick-fix method of drugs and alcohol for relief. However, for long-term results a more radical approach should be sought.*

The yogic scriptures state that pure relaxation is experienced when not only the body, but also the mind and spirit, are entirely relaxed. This degree of deep relaxation is achieved through training and awareness. Like the trident of the Hindu deity Shiva, yoga uses a three-pronged approach.

## I. Physical

Yoga asanas actually promote relaxation in the muscles. Try lying in the Relax Pose (Savasana Pose, shown right) both before and after ashtanga practice and experience the differences. Generally, the Relax Pose is the last pose performed, right at the end of your practice, at which point the muscles are completely relaxed. However, it can also be used before you begin your practice, along with breath control, in order to release any superficial tensions from the day.

## 2. Mental

To aid physical relaxation, Laya yoga (or visualization) is performed. Yogic sutras speak of imagining the body filled with divine bliss or nectar, but there are many positive images that you can evoke. It is important to find one that feels comfortable for you. Rather than visualization, some people prefer to scan the entire body, starting from the feet and consciously letting go of each area. Others benefit from simply experiencing the silence around them.

## 3. Spiritual

Spiritual relaxation is the hardest to achieve and requires a very deep letting go, relinquishing control of both body and mind, and putting your trust in a higher source. By deeply letting go for a few moments you can experience a profound inner peace and silence.

# RELAX POSE

■ It is essential to finish each asana practice with the Relax Pose (Savasana) for a minimum of 10 minutes. This allows the body to rebalance itself after the effects of the poses.

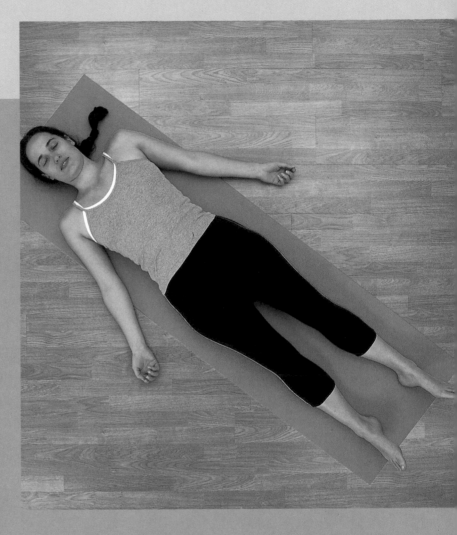

■ Lie on your back with your head and spine in alignment. Your arms should fall about 10 inches/ 25 cm from your body, with your palms facing upward.

■ Your legs should be about hip-width apart and your feet relaxed, so that they fall naturally to the sides.

■ Slowly roll your neck from side to side, then tuck your chin in slightly and extend through the back of your neck.

■ Consciously release any tension that remains in your body (especially your face and jaws). If you experience any tightness in your body, you can

tense the muscles in that area, then release them.

■ Once your body is relaxed, bring your attention to your breathing. Ujjayi breathing should be stopped at this point and replaced by silent natural breathing. As you exhale, imagine any remaining tension leaving your body; as you inhale, imagine vital new energy entering it. Try not to let the mind wander. If it does, gently bring it back to your breathing.

■ After 10 minutes start to bring the awareness back into your body. Raise your arms over your head and take a deep stretch, from your toes to fingertips. Then roll over onto your left side and stay there for a few moments before getting up.

# Safety first

*The purpose of asana practice is to keep the body clear of physical obstacles such as disease. The yoga poses in the primary Ashtanga series specifically aim to detoxify and realign the musculoskeletal system.*

During practice of the primary series, various weaknesses in the body may come to light. This is an inevitable result of the purification process. Guruji has a very hard-line approach to any pains that arise through practice, which is to carry on working through the problem. This approach can be quite shocking to Westerners. However, I have personally witnessed many miraculous results from practitioners continuing with their yoga through even the most severe injuries.

From my own experience of working with hereditary back problems, and from my knowledge acquired through other systems of yoga, I prefer a gentler approach.

Pain and injury offer us a unique opportunity to broaden our understanding of ourselves – we are given an insight into our own limitations and into how to work with or around them. In the interests of safety, it is best to observe the following advice below and opposite.

## IN CASE OF INJURY

■ If a muscle or ligament is torn during practice, put some ice on it immediately to reduce the swelling.

■ Avoid any poses that aggravate an injury. A good yoga instructor should be able to give you a series of remedial poses to speed recovery.

■ In the case of a leg or wrist injury, use a support stocking during practice until the injury has healed.

# SAFETY TIPS

Always use a non-slip yoga mat, so that there is no danger of slipping during your practice.

Do not wear tight or restrictive clothing, or any jewelry that may restrict the blood circulation.

For Ashtanga practice it is especially important to work in a warm environment. In the cold, the muscles contract and are far more prone to injury.

If you have any medical problems, seek advice from your teacher and from your physician before practicing.

Do not force yourself into any particular pose; only go as far as your own capacity allows.

It is important to keep breathing, even during the most complex poses – often when we are trying to do a difficult task, we tend to hold our breath without realizing it.

■ Do not practice asana after long periods of sunbathing.

■ Do not practice inverted (upside-down) poses if you are suffering from high blood pressure, or during menstruation.

■ If you experience exhaustion, then your practice has been too prolonged for your current constitution.

■ Pain that arises during practice should be only temporary. If it becomes persistent, then you may be practicing incorrectly. If you experience excessive pain in a pose, stop it immediately.

# CHAPTER ONE
# Warming up

The Salute to the Sun *(Surya Namaskar)* sequence is reputed to stabilize the mind and bring contentment. Symbolically, the act of prostration is a devotional one, representing the surrender of the self to the universal spirit or higher consciousness, which is said to be within – as well as outside of – ourselves. The movements are best performed while repeating a specific mantra to help focus the mind. There are two levels of Salute to the Sun (A and B). Together they form an excellent warm-up routine, which limbers the spine, creates internal heat in the body, and prepares it for the rest of the sequence. Each full sequence should be repeated five times.

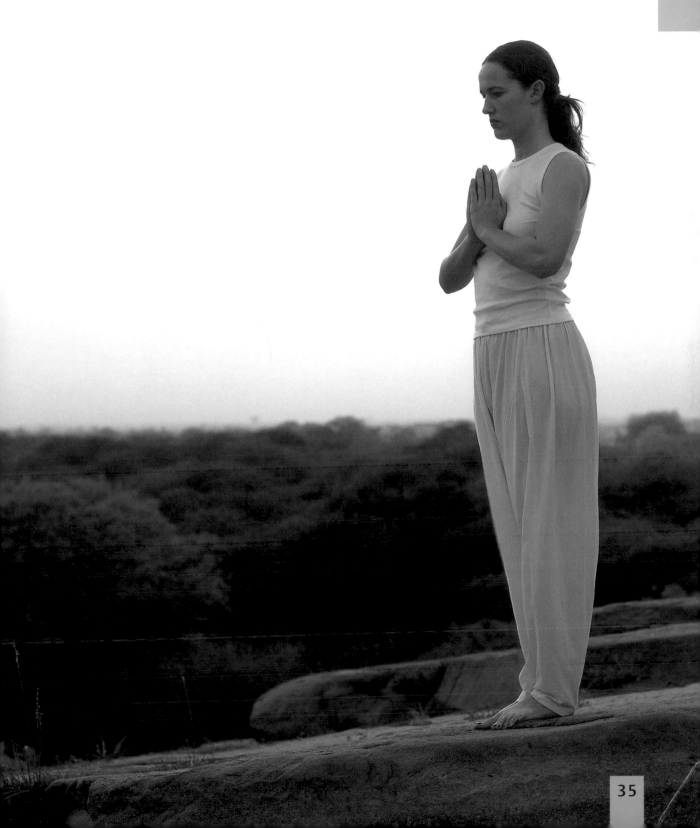

# Salute to the Sun (A)
## Surya Namaskar (A)

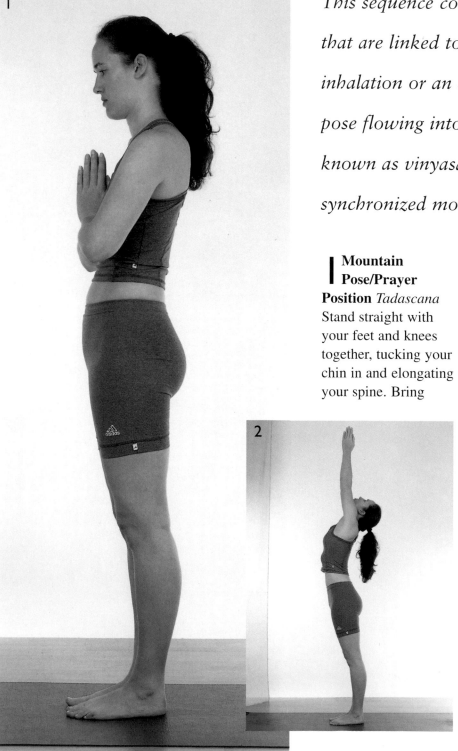

*This sequence consists of 11 poses that are linked together by an inhalation or an exhalation – one pose flowing into the next. This is known as vinyasa, or breath-synchronized movement.*

**1 Mountain Pose/Prayer Position** *Tadascana*
Stand straight with your feet and knees together, tucking your chin in and elongating your spine. Bring your palms together at the center of your chest, and focus your attention on your breathing. This is an effective pose, which helps to center the mind and body.

**2 Hands Above the Head**
*Urdhva Hastasana U*
**Inhale:** raise your hands outward, drawing a large circle in the air until your palms are touching again, over your head, in the Prayer Position. Lean your head back and look up toward your thumbs.

3

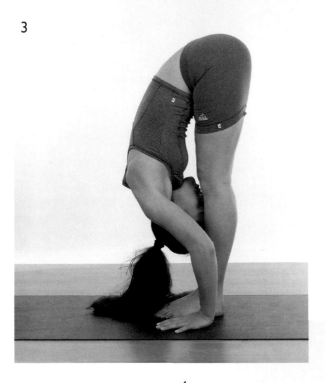

## 3 Forward Bend
*Uttanasana*

**Exhale:** releasing your breath slowly, bend forward from the hips, keeping your back straight. Bring your hands down to the floor on either side of your feet. Place your head between your knees.

**Beginners:** if it is not possible to touch the floor with your legs straight, then you can bend your knees. Once in this position, try to extend your legs by lifting your buttocks and straightening your legs through the backs of your knees.

4

## 4 Head Up
*Uttasana*

**Inhale:** as you slowly inhale, lift your head up, keeping your hands flat on the floor. Look up toward your "third eye" in the middle of your forehead. Straightening your arms, make your lower back concave and extend toward your tailbone.

**Beginners:** come up onto your fingertips.

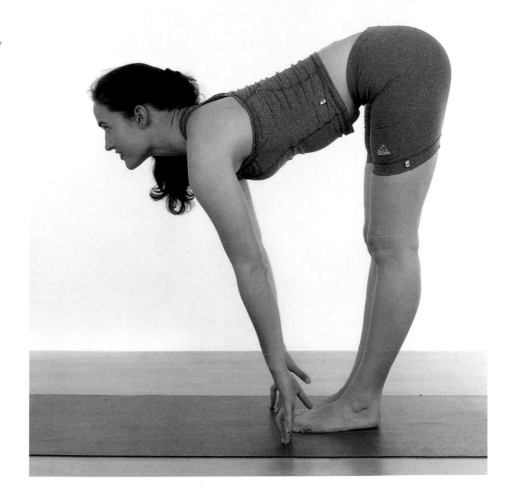

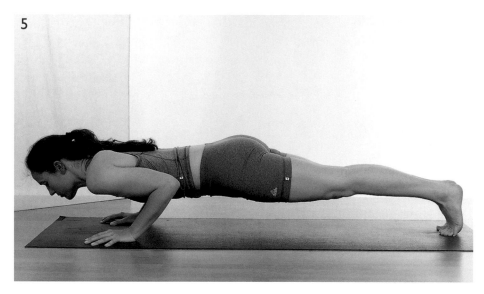

**5 Four-Limbed Stick** *Caturanga Dandasana*
**Exhale:** using the strength of your hands, jump back into a press-up position or straight line (see p. 41), with just your toes and the palms of your hands touching the floor. Your elbows should be tucked in close to your sides, holding your body parallel to the floor. Your feet should be hip-width apart.

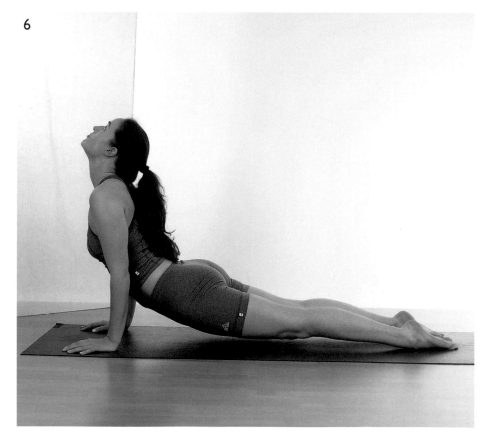

**6 Upward Dog** *Urdhva Mukha Svanasana*
**Inhale:** roll over your toes onto the tops of your feet. Bring your chest forward and up through your arms, rolling your shoulders over and back. Arch your back and look up. Try to keep your upper legs raised off the floor.

■ **Beginners:** you may find it difficult to keep the legs raised, but this will come with practice.

## 7 Downward Dog
*Adho Mukha Svanasana*

**Exhale:** pushing into the palms of your hands, roll back over your toes onto the soles of your feet. Take your heels down toward the floor and pull your hips up into the air. Keep your hands in line with each other and your feet parallel. Your arms should be straight, with the inner elbows facing each other. Tuck your chin down, look toward your navel, and take either five or eight long breaths.

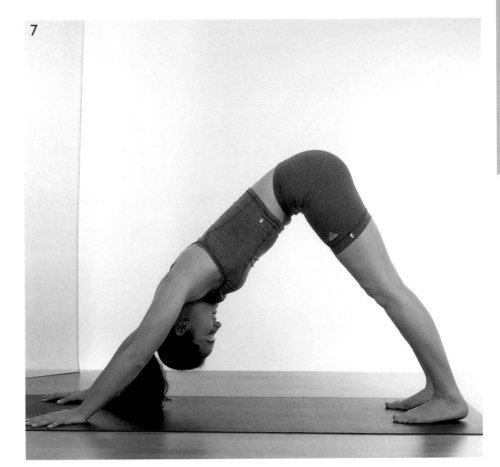

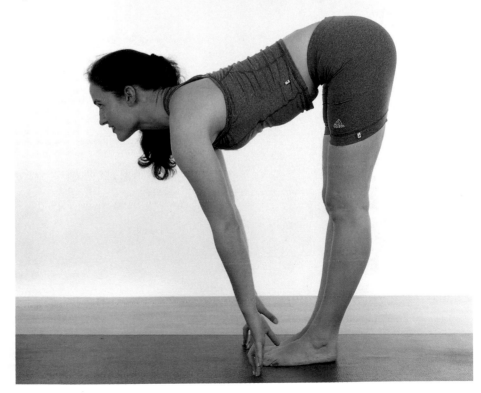

## 8 Forward Bend/Head Up
*Uttasana*

**Inhale:** jump into a Forward Bend with the head up (Step 4).

■ **Beginners:** you can step the feet forward between the hands one at a time.

9

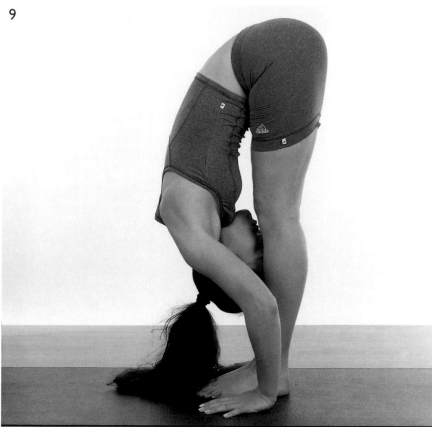

**9 Forward Bend**
*Uttanasana*
**Exhale:** take the head down toward the knees.

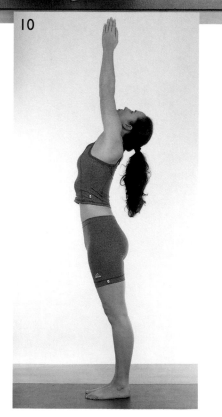

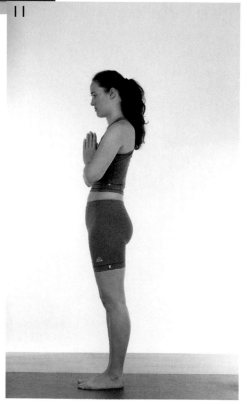

**10 Hands Above the Head**
*Urdhva Hastasana U*
**Inhale:** stand tall, then bring your hands together in the Prayer Position over your head.

**11 Mountain Pose Prayer Position**
*Tadascana*
**Exhale:** draw your hands down in a straight line to the center of your chest.

Repeat the whole sequence five times.

# HOW TO ACHIEVE THE JUMP-BACK

Jumping produces agility in body and mind, though initially it takes practice.

■ First, bring the weight of the body forward onto the palms of your hands.

■ Then jump the feet up and back in a straight line, so that you land on your toes, which should be hip-width apart. Bend your elbows close to your sides at the same time, so that you land in the correct position. If this is too difficult, initially you can jump back keeping your arms straight.

■ Next, slowly lower yourself into a press-up position in a straight line.

■ For a beginner or for anyone with back problems, do not jump back; instead, step your feet back one at a time and then gently lower yourself into a press-up position.

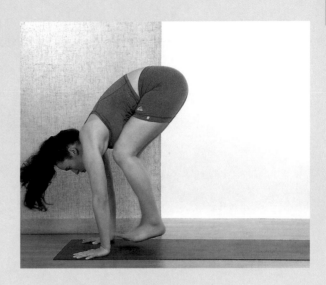

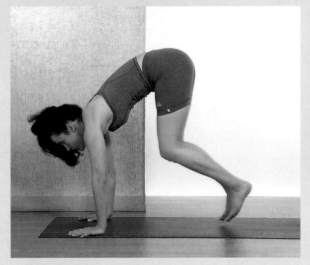

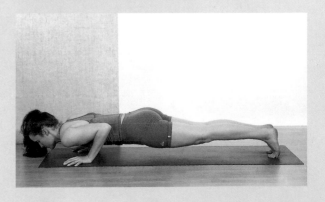

# fast index to Salute to the Sun (A)

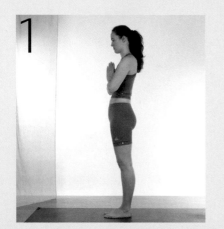

Mountain Pose/Prayer Position

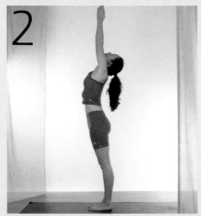

Hands Above the Head

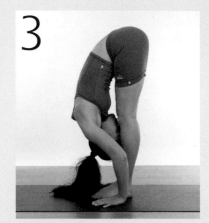

Forward Bend

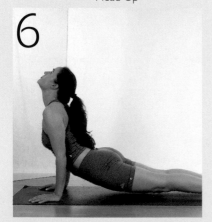

Head Up

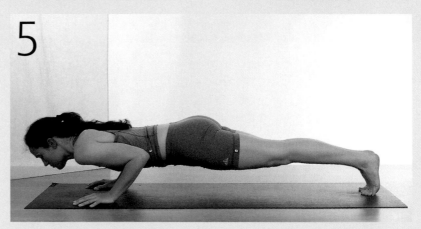

Four-Limbed Stick

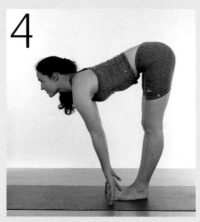

Upward Dog

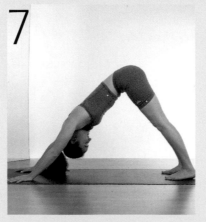

Downward Dog

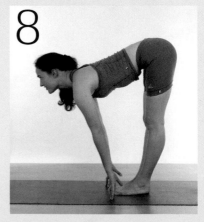

Forward Bend/Head Up

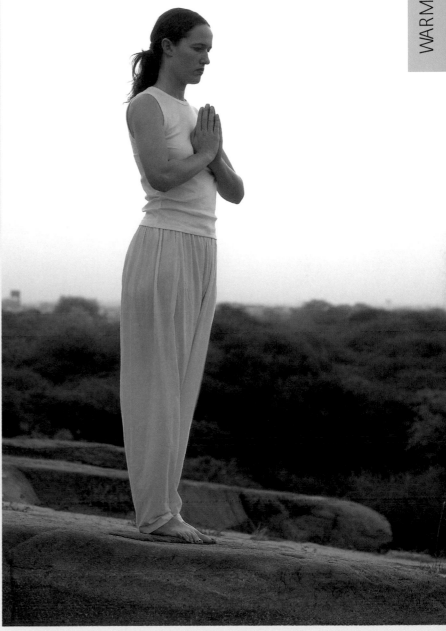

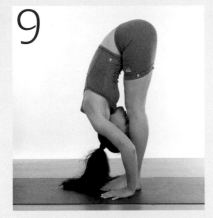

**9**

Forward Bend

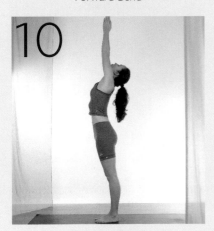

**10**

Hands Above the Head

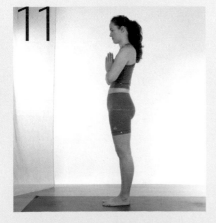

**11**

Mountain Pose/Prayer Position

# HELPFUL HINT

While practicing Salute to the Sun (A), most beginners will experience stiffness caused by a build-up of muscular tension. To avoid straining your body, study each posture, then practice them in sequence very slowly in time with your breathing. If you get exhausted or breathless, rest between each cycle. With practice, the poses will become fluid and pain-free.

# Salute to the Sun (B)
## Surya Namaskar (B)

*This is a more challenging sequence, with 17 poses flowing from one to another. Start from the Even Pose (Samasthitih), which is a neutral, yet alert, standing pose, with the feet together and your hands by your sides.*

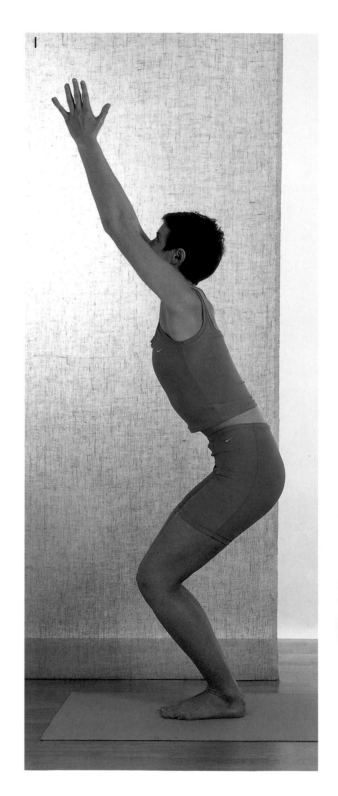

**| Powerful Pose**
*Utkatasana*
**Inhale**: as you lift your hands into the Prayer Position (see p. 36) above your head, simultaneously bend your legs, as if you are about to sit down. When your legs are bent at a 60° angle, hold the position and lift up through your arms, while pressing your heels firmly into the floor. Grip your knees together and lean the weight of your body back onto your heels. Keep lifting your back so your trunk does not lean too far forward. Lift your head and look up at your thumbs.

**2** **Forward Bend**
*Uttanasana*
**Exhale:** lean into a
Forward Bend, taking
your head between
your knees as in
Salute to the Sun A,
Step 3 (see p. 37).

2

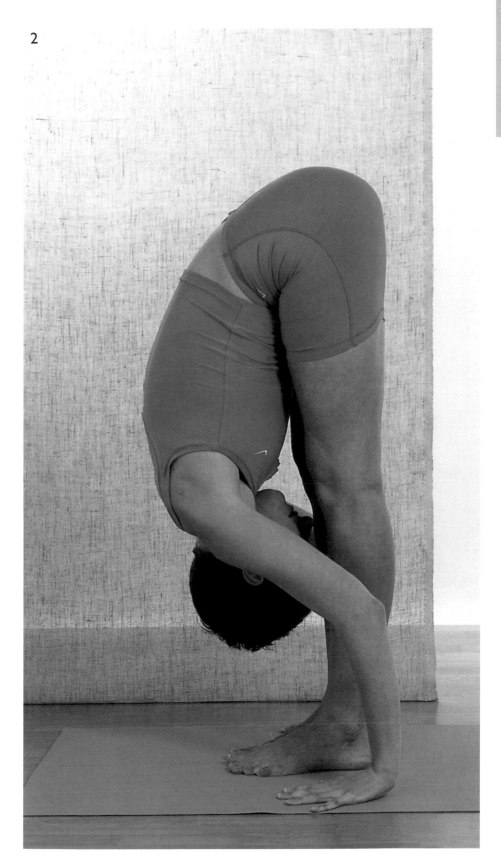

3

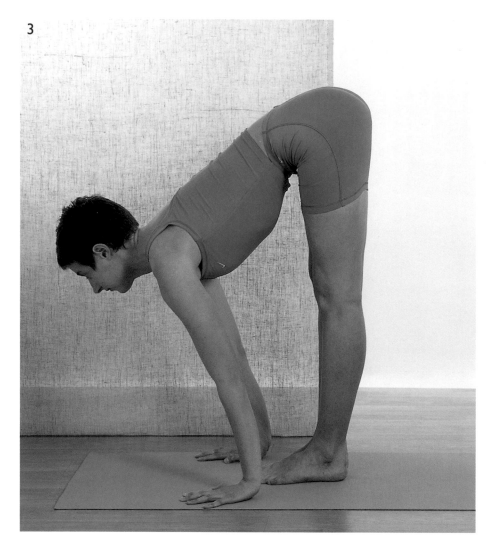

### 3 Forward Bend/Head Up
*Uttasana*
**Inhale:** as you lift your head and trunk, straighten your arms, while keeping your hands flat on the floor. Look toward your "third eye."

### 4 Four-Limbed Stick
*Caturanga Dandasana*
**Exhale:** either jump or step back into the press-up position.

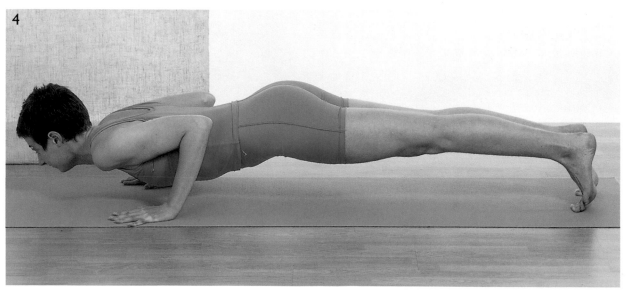

4

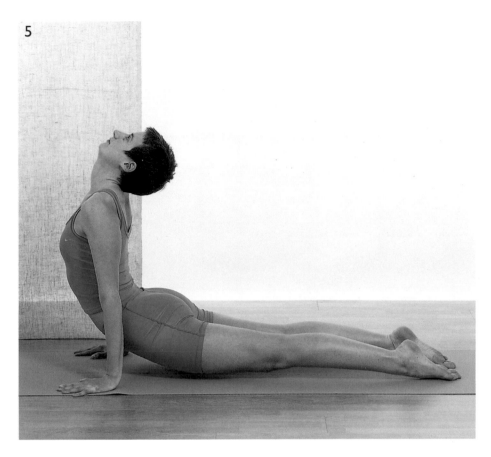

**5**

### 5 Upward Dog
*Urdhva Mukha Svanasana*

**Inhale:** push into the palms of your hands and roll over onto the tops of your feet, keeping your thighs and knees off the floor. Lift your chest, bend your back, and look up toward your "third eye".

### 6 Downward Dog
*Adho Mukha Svanasana*

**Exhale:** push back through your hands, roll back over your toes onto the soles of your feet, and take your heels toward the floor. Straighten your arms, lifting away from the palms toward your raised buttocks. Keep your thigh muscles contracted. Bend your head and look toward your navel.

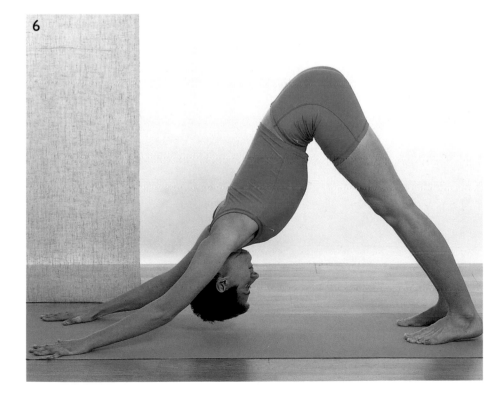

**6**

7a

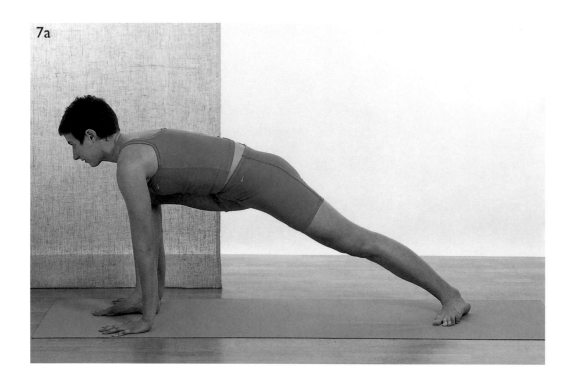

# 7 Warrior Pose
*Virabhadrasana*

7b

**Inhale:** step your right leg forward, taking the foot between your hands (see 7a). Raise your trunk and lift your arms into the Prayer Position above your head, keeping your arms straight and your shoulders down. Your right leg should stay at a 90° angle, with your thigh parallel to the floor. Your left leg should remain straight. Your hips should face forward. Lift your trunk up, expanding the chest. Look up toward your thumbs (see 7b).

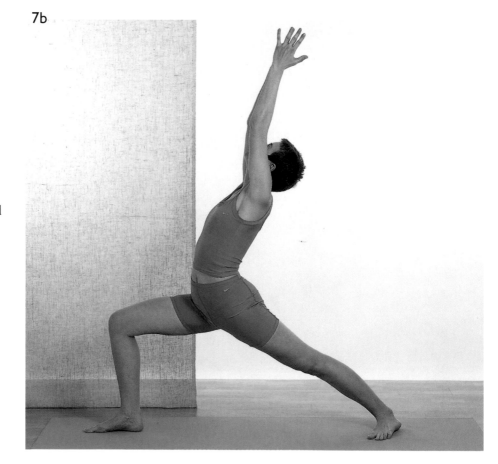

# COMPLETING THE SEQUENCE

See the fast index (overleaf) for a visual reminder of every pose.

To complete Salute to the Sun B you need to repeat combinations of some of the poses you have just tried.

**8** From the **Warrior Pose** (Step 7), go to the **Four-Limbed Stick** pose (Step 4). **Exhale:** bend forward, putting your hands on either side of your right foot, then take your right foot back so that both feet are in line. Lower your body into a press-up position.

**9** Go into the **Upward Dog** pose (Step 5). **Inhale:** roll over your toes, straighten your arms, and lift your chest, looking upward.

**10** Now go into the **Downward Dog** (Step 6). **Exhale:** press into your palms and roll backward over your toes, taking your heels toward the floor. Staighten your arms, raise your buttocks, draw in your stomach, and look toward your navel.

**11** Repeat the **Warrior Pose** (Step 7). **Inhale:** step your right foot forward between your hands. Lift your trunk and raise your arms together in the Prayer Position over your head. Look up toward your thumbs.

**12** Repeat the **Four-Limbed Stick** (Step 4). **Exhale:** step your left foot back in line with your right, then lower yourself into a press-up position.

**13** Repeat the **Upward Dog** (Step 5). **Inhale:** roll over your toes, straighten your arms, lift your chest, and look at your "third eye."

**14** Repeat the **Downward Dog** (Step 6). **Exhale:** press into your palms and roll backward over your toes, taking your heels toward the floor. Straighten your arms, lift your buttocks, tighten your stomach muscles, and look toward your navel.

**15** Repeat the **Forward Bend/Head Up** (Step 3). **Inhale:** jump both feet together between your hands, keeping your head raised as you do so.

**16** Repeat the **Forward Bend** (Step 2).

**Exhale:** take your head down to your knees.

**17** Repeat the **Powerful Pose** (Step 1). **Inhale:** bend your knees and lift your torso from the hips. Raise your arms above your head and take your hands into the **Prayer Position,** looking up toward your thumbs.

Then return to a standing position by lowering your arms and straightening your knees. Repeat the whole sequence five times.

# fast index to Salute to the Sun (B)

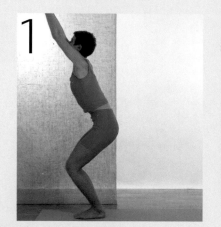

**1**

Powerful Pose

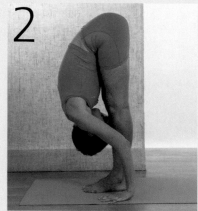

**2**

Forward Bend

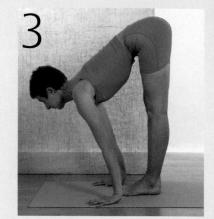

**3**

Forward Bend/Head Up

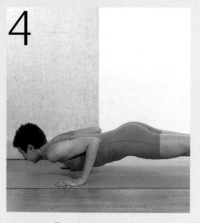

**4**

Four-Limbed Stick

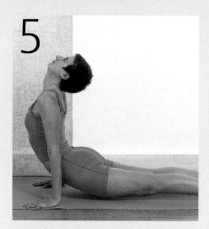

**5**

Upward Dog

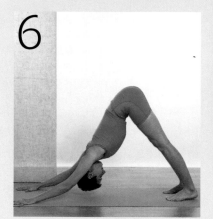

**6**

Downward Dog

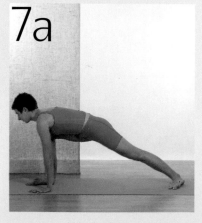

**7a**

Warrior Pose

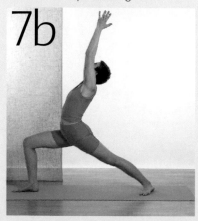

**7b**

Warrior Pose

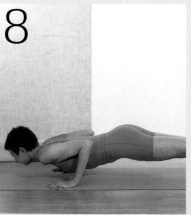

**8**

Four-Limbed Stick

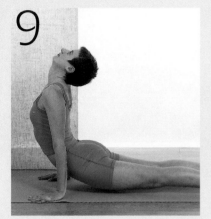

**9**

Upward Dog

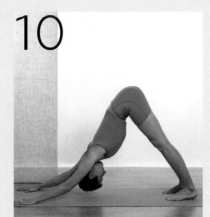

**10**

Downward Dog

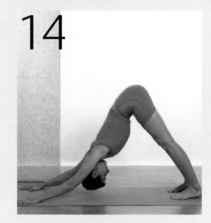

**11**

Warrior Pose

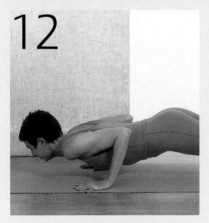

**12**

Four-Limbed Stick

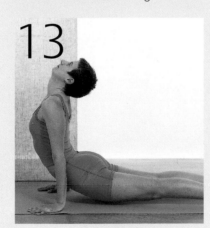

**13**

Upward Dog

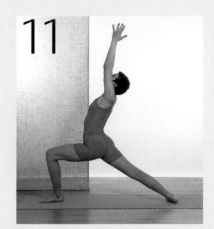

**14**

Downward Dog

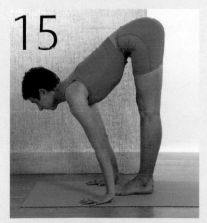

**15**

Forward Bend/Head Up

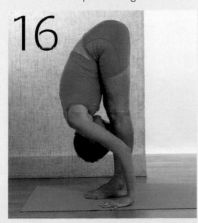

**16**

Forward Bend

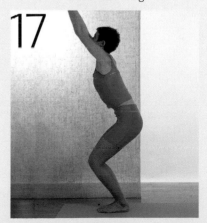

**17**

Powerful Pose

CHAPTER TWO

# Standing poses

The first standing poses are fundamental to all forms of yoga, helping to build strength in the legs and bring suppleness to the spine. The standing poses help revitalize the whole physical system, bringing new oxygen and blood to the vital organs. These poses are particularly curative for people who are suffering from rheumatism or from general aches and pains in the joints. Beginners should hold the poses for five breaths, although more advanced practitioners can hold them for eight breaths. Between each standing pose, jump back into the Even Pose – this is simply standing straight with your hands by your sides.

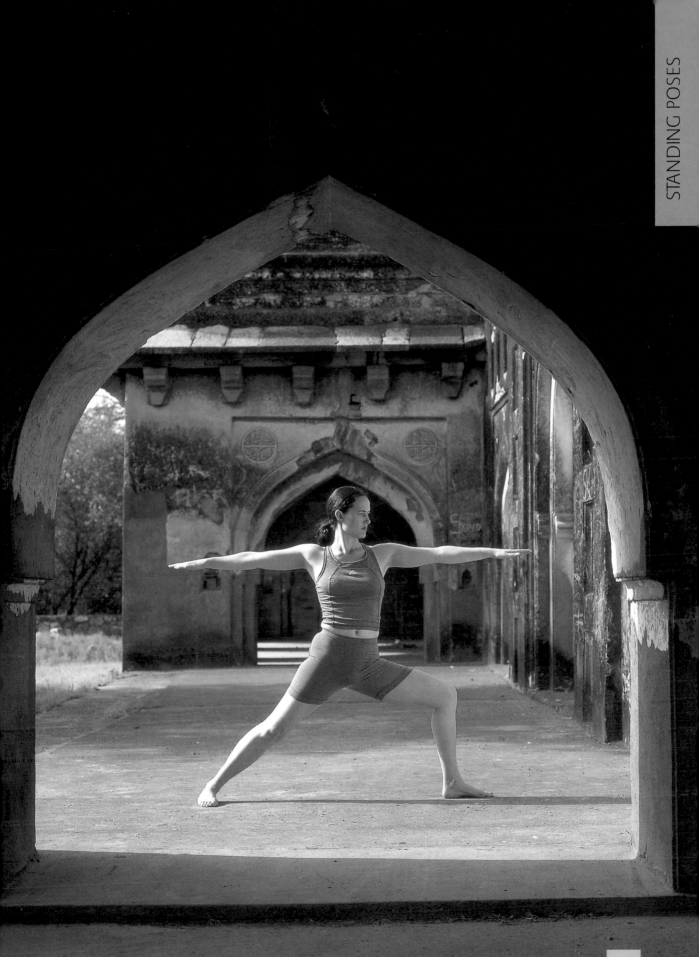

# Standing poses

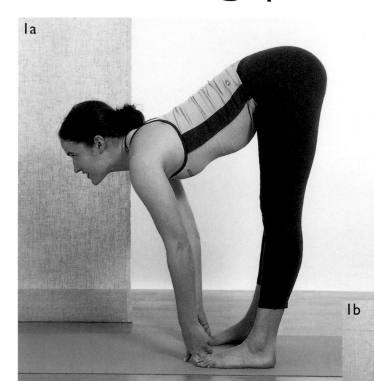

la

1b

*The first six poses promote flexibility in the spine and prepare the body for the more difficult poses that follow; they also purify the digestive organs.*

**Forward Bend A**
*Padangushtsana*
Adopt the Even Pose – stand straight with your hands by your sides, feet together, and your big toes and ankle bones touching.
**Inhale:** jump the feet 6 inches/15 cm apart.
**Warning:** If you suffer from knee or back problems, then step the legs apart.
**Inhale:** expand your chest, pull in your stomach muscles, and elongate your spine.
**Exhale:** bend forward from your hips and take hold of your two big toes with your thumbs and two fore-fingers. Your weight should be balanced over the center of your feet, with your legs perpendicular.
**Beginners:** if you cannot reach your big toes, hold behind the ankles or as close as you can reach.
**Inhale:** lift your head, straighten your arms, and look up (see 1a). Keep your legs active and strong, with your thigh muscles lifting up and toward each other. This movement broadens the hips and allows you to go deeper into the pose.
**Exhale:** take your head down between your knees, and bend your elbows out to the sides (see 1b).

This is the full asana. Hold for the duration of five long breaths.
**Inhale:** with your legs straight, raise your trunk and return to a standing position.
**Warning:** If you have any lower back pain, then slightly bend the knees as you lift yourself up.

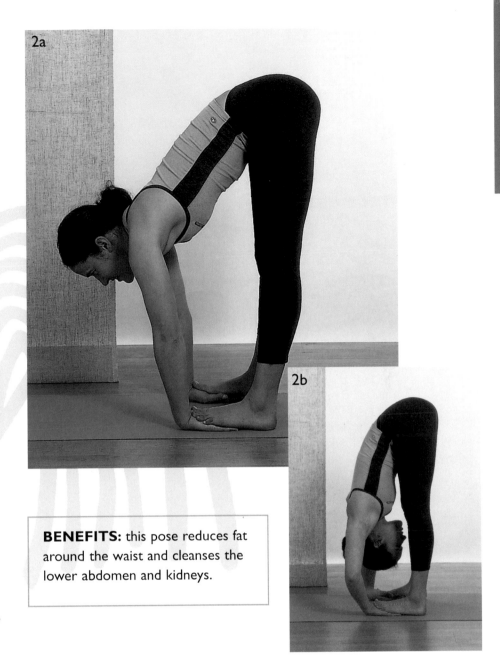

2a

2b

## 2 Forward Bend B
*Padahastasana*

Stand in the Even Pose, so your hands are by your sides, your feet are together, and your big toes and ankle bones are touching.

**Inhale:** lift your chest and elongate your spine.

**Exhale:** bend forward from the hips, and place your upward palms under the soles of your feet (see 2a).

■ **Beginners:** stretch down as far as possible and hold behind the legs.

**Inhale:** straighten your arms and lift your head, looking up toward the "third eye" Be aware of the elongation of your spine. Draw up your kneecaps.

**Exhale:** bend your elbows out to the sides and take your head down between your knees (see 2b). Hold for five long breaths.

**Inhale:** release your hands and lift your trunk upright.

**BENEFITS:** this pose reduces fat around the waist and cleanses the lower abdomen and kidneys.

## HAND-HOLD TECHNIQUES

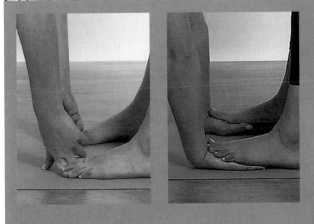

■ Hold the big toe as in Step 1, with index finger, middle finger, and thumb, (left). This stimulates the pituitary gland, and the throat. In Step 2 (above), the palms are placed under the soles, setting up an energy circuit in the body (see p. 26).

55

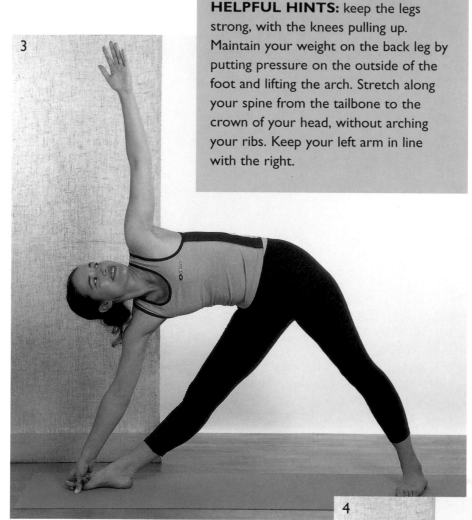

3

**HELPFUL HINTS:** keep the legs strong, with the knees pulling up. Maintain your weight on the back leg by putting pressure on the outside of the foot and lifting the arch. Stretch along your spine from the tailbone to the crown of your head, without arching your ribs. Keep your left arm in line with the right.

## 4 Reversed Triangle

*Parivita Trikonasana*
**Exhale:** turn the right foot out by 90°, and the left foot in at a 60° angle. Lift your arms out to the sides. Turn your hips, torso, and head to face the right leg. Bend forward and down, and place your left hand, palm down, on the outside of your right foot. Turn your head to look up at your right thumb.
**Breath:** hold for five steady breaths.
**Inhale:** lift and rotate your body back to the center. Repeat on the other side.

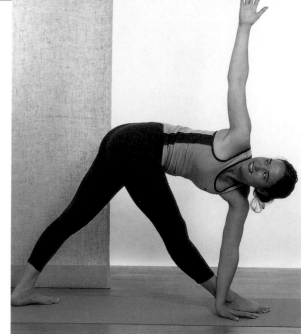

4

## 3 Extended Triangle

*Utthita Trikonasana*
Stand in the Even Pose, with your hands by your sides and your feet together.
**Inhale:** jump the feet 3–4 feet/1–1.2 m apart.
**Exhale:** as you turn your right foot out by 90°, turn your left foot in slightly. Rotate your right leg from the thigh, but keep your hips facing forward. Raise your arms to the sides to shoulder height, with palms facing the floor. Then stretch to the right, keeping the torso facing forward, and take your right hand down to hold the right big toe, and look up at your left thumb. This is the full asana, so hold for five deep breaths.
**Inhale:** with a deep inhalation come to the center. Repeat on the other side.

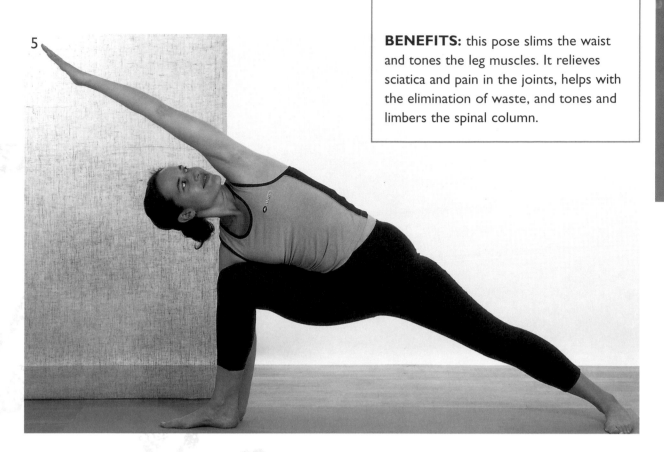

5

## 5 Extended Sideways Pose

*Utthita Parsvakonasana*

**Inhale:** jump the feet 4–5 feet/1.2–1.5 m apart, with your arms outstretched.

**Exhale:** turn your right foot out by 90° and your left foot in slightly. Bend the right knee until your thigh forms a right-angle with your calf. Lean over the right leg, with your right hand on the outside of the right foot. Stretch your left arm up and over your head to draw a diagonal line. Look up.

**Breath:** hold for five breaths.

**Inhale:** come back to the center. Repeat on the other side.

## 6 Spread-Leg Pose A *Prasarita Padottanasana A*

**Inhale:** jump the feet 4–5 feet/1.2–1.5 m apart and parallel.

**Exhale:** bend forward and drop your hands to the floor below your shoulders.

**Inhale:** look up and feel the stretch in your whole spine.

**Exhale:** take your hands back, in line with your feet, and place the crown of your head between your hands.

**Breath:** hold for five long breaths.

**Inhale:** straighten the arms and take your head up. Look to the "third eye."

**Exhale:** and hold.

**Inhale:** come up to the center.

6

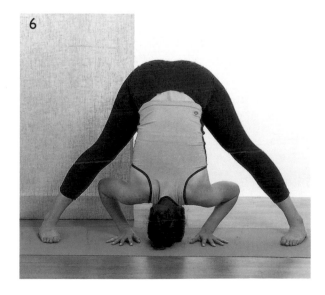

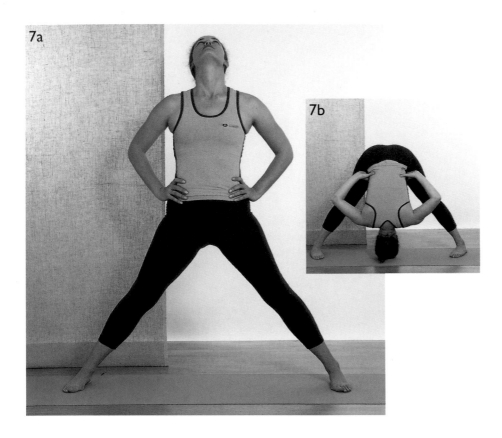

7a

7b

## 7 Spread-Leg Pose B *Prasarita Padottanasana B*

**Inhale:** jump the feet 4–5 feet/1.2–1.5 m apart, with open arms.
**Exhale:** place your hands on your waist.
**Inhale:** look up (see 7a).
**Exhale:** bend forward, taking your head to the floor (see 7b).
**Breath:** hold for five long breaths.
**Inhale:** come up.
**Exhale:** jump the feet together into the Even Pose, standing straight with your hands by your sides.

## 8 Spread-Leg Pose C *Prasarita Padottanasana C*

**Inhale:** jump the feet so they are 4–5 feet/ 1.2–1.5 m apart, with open arms.
**Exhale:** interlock your fingers behind your back.
**Inhale:** straighten your arms; look up.
**Exhale:** bend forward and place the crown of your head on the floor. Allow your arms to drop naturally to the floor.
**Breath:** rest for five breaths.
**Inhale:** come up.

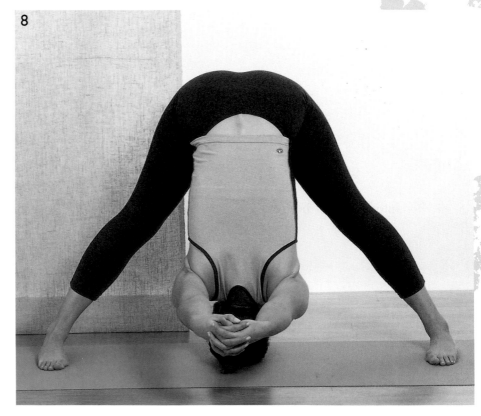

8

## 9 Spread-Leg Pose D *Prasarita Padottanasana D*

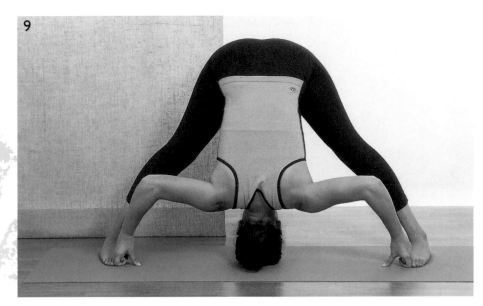

**Inhale:** jump the feet 4–5 feet/1.2–1.5 m apart, with your hands on your waist.

**Exhale:** bend forward and hold both the big toes with your thumbs and two forefingers.

**Inhale:** straighten your arms; look up.

**Exhale:** bend your elbows out to the sides and take the crown of your head to the floor, between your feet.

**Breath:** hold for five long breaths.

**Inhale:** straighten your arms; look up.

**Exhale:** rest.

**Inhale:** come back up into the Even Pose, standing straight with your feet together and hands by your sides.

■ **Beginners:** if you cannot take your head to the floor, widen the legs by 1 ft/3 cm.

■ **Advanced:** if your head reaches the floor easily, bring your feet closer together.

## 10 Sideways Extension

*Parsvottanasana*
*Note that this pose should begin on the right side, but is shown here on the left side for variation.*

**Inhale:** jump the feet 3 feet/1 m apart. Put your hands into the Prayer Position behind your back between the shoulder blades. Turn your left foot out by 90° and your right foot by about 60° and swivel your hips and upper body to face the left leg. Open your upper chest, take your head back, and look up.

**Exhale:** bend from the hips, over your left leg, taking your chin down to the shin.

**Breath:** hold this pose for five breaths.

**Inhale:** on a deep inhalation, lift your body up and back to the center.

**Exhale:** turn your feet to the right side and repeat the pose.

■ **Beginners:** if you cannot put your hands in the Prayer Position, then hold your elbows and bend as far forward as possible.

**BENEFITS:** this pose strengthens and tones the leg muscles, slims the waist, and removes mucus from the respiratory tract.

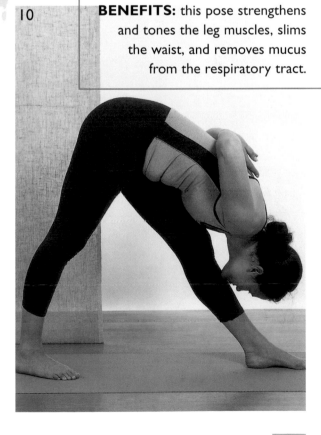

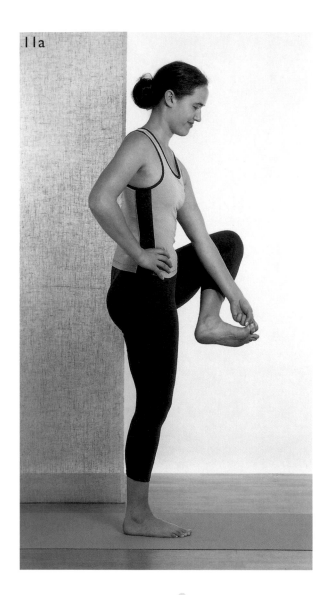

11a

**Breath:** hold for five breaths.

**Inhale:** lift your head while keeping hold of the big toe (see 11b).

**Exhale:** rotate the leg out to the left side, keeping your hips level. Look away from the left leg over your right shoulder (see 11c).

**Breath:** hold for five breaths.

**Inhale:** rotate the left leg forward.

**Exhale:** lift the leg as high as possible and take your head to the knee.

**Inhale:** let go of the leg, but keep it raised with the strength of the leg muscles. Put your left hand on your waist, draw in your stomach muscles, and squeeze with your hands (see 11d).

**Breath:** hold this position for five breaths.

**Exhale:** lower the leg to the floor.

**Inhale:** lift the right leg and catch hold of the big toe, then repeat all the movements on the other side.

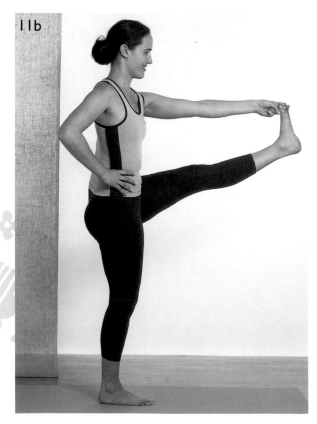

11b

**11 Thumb-to-Foot Pose**

*Utthita Hasta Padangusthasana*
*Note that this pose should begin on the right side, but is shown here on the left side for variation.* Stand in the Even Pose, with hands by your sides and your feet touching.

**Inhale:** bend your left leg and take hold of the big toe with the thumb and forefingers of your left hand. Keep your right hand on your waist (see 11a).

**Exhale:** straighten the left leg and take your head toward the knee. Keep the leg straight and the muscles taut.

**HELPFUL HINTS:** to assist your balance, pick a spot on the floor in front of you to look at, which focuses your attention. Keep the big toe of your standing foot pushing into the floor and your thigh muscles active.

11c

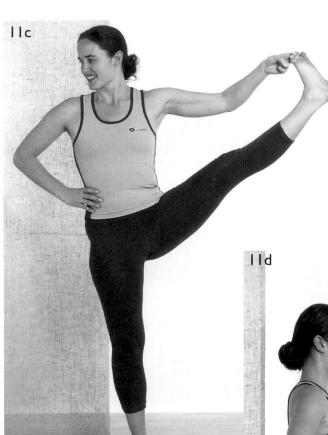

11d

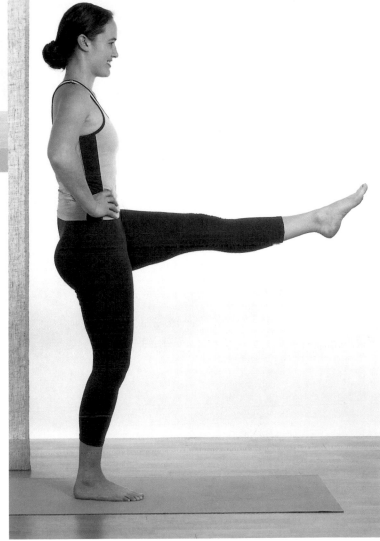

■ **Beginners:** initially you will need the help of a teacher or partner to hold the raised leg steady. You can also practice by placing your raised foot on a high ledge until you get your balance.

**BENEFITS:** this pose strengthens the leg muscles and increases steadiness and poise. It also stimulates the nerves in the tailbone and tones the kidneys.

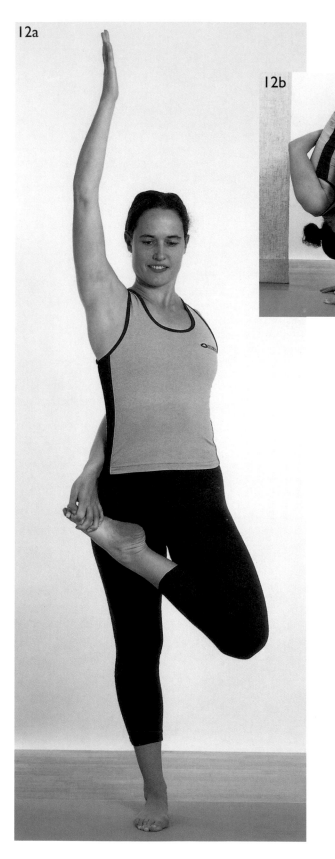

12a

12b

## 12 Half-Bound Lotus Stretch

*Ardha Baddha Padmottanasana*
*Note that this pose should begin on the right side, but is shown here on the left side for variation.*
Stand in the Even Pose, with your hands by your sides and your feet together.
**Inhale:** take the ankle of your left foot and place it at the top of your right thigh. Rotate the left leg, so your left knee points toward the floor, in line with your right knee. Bind the pose by swinging your left arm behind your back and grabbing hold of the left big toe. Stand tall with your right arm raised (see 12a).
**Exhale:** bend forward from your hips, and take your right hand to the outside of your right foot. Take your chin toward your shin (see 12b).
**Breath:** hold for five breaths.
**Inhale:** come up to a standing position.
**Exhale:** release the left leg.
**Inhale:** lift and bend the other leg; repeat on the other side.
■ **Beginners**: this is a tough pose for beginners, so practice 12a only, then proceed from there.

**HELPFUL HINTS:** if you cannot reach your big toe, try bending forward and then taking hold of it. If you have a problem coming up, or have lower back problems, slightly bend the standing leg and then come up.

## 13 Uneven Pose
*Utkatasana*

Stand in the Even Pose, with your hands by your sides and your feet together.

**Inhale:** the first few movements are the same as Salute to the Sun A (see p. 36). Raise your arms over your head into the Prayer Position, then look up toward your thumbs, as shown.

**Exhale:** bend forward and place your hands on the outside of, and in line with, your feet.

**Inhale:** lift your head and look up to the "third eye."

**Exhale:** jump back into the Four-Limbed Stick (see p. 38), with just hands and toes touching the floor.

**Inhale:** straighten your arms and press into your palms as you roll over onto the tops of your feet for the Upward Dog pose (see p. 38).

**Exhale:** raise your buttocks, press into your palms, and roll backward over your toes onto the soles of

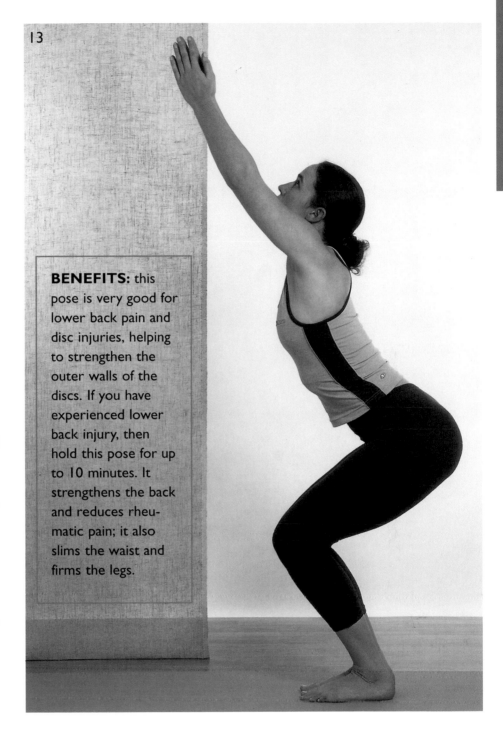

13

**BENEFITS:** this pose is very good for lower back pain and disc injuries, helping to strengthen the outer walls of the discs. If you have experienced lower back injury, then hold this pose for up to 10 minutes. It strengthens the back and reduces rheumatic pain; it also slims the waist and firms the legs.

your feet, into Downward Dog (see p. 39).

**Inhale:** jump your feet forward between your hands, bend your knees, and raise your arms above your head into the Prayer Position. Look up toward your thumbs, as shown.

**Breath:** hold for five even breaths.

**Exhale:** bend forward, place your hands on the outside of your feet, straighten your legs, and take your head down between your knees. Repeat the jump-back series, then return to a standing position.

14a

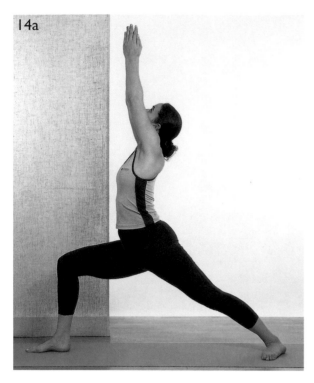

14b

14c

# 14 Warrior Pose A

*Virabhadrasana A*

**Inhale:** the first movements are Steps 1, 2, and 3 of Salute to the Sun A (see pp. 36–37). From the Even Pose (standing straight with feet together and hands by your sides) raise your arms over your head and bend you knees. Look up to your thumbs.

**Exhale:** bend forward, place your palms on the floor alongside your feet, straighten your legs, and take your head down between your knees.

**Inhale:** look up.

**Exhale:** jump back into the Four-Limbed Stick (see p. 38).

**Inhale:** move into the Upward Dog (see p. 38).

**Exhale:** move into the Downward Dog (see p. 39).

**Inhale:** step the right foot forward between your hands. Raise your trunk and lift your arms into the Prayer Position, with arms straight and shoulders down (see 14a). Keep the right leg at 90°, with your thigh parallel to the floor; keep your left leg straight, with your hips facing forward. Lift your trunk up and expand your chest. Look up toward your thumbs.

**Breath:** hold for five long breaths.

**Inhale:** straighten the front leg, turn to the center (see 14b) then turn to the left side and repeat the pose (see 14c). Move into Warrior Pose B.

15a

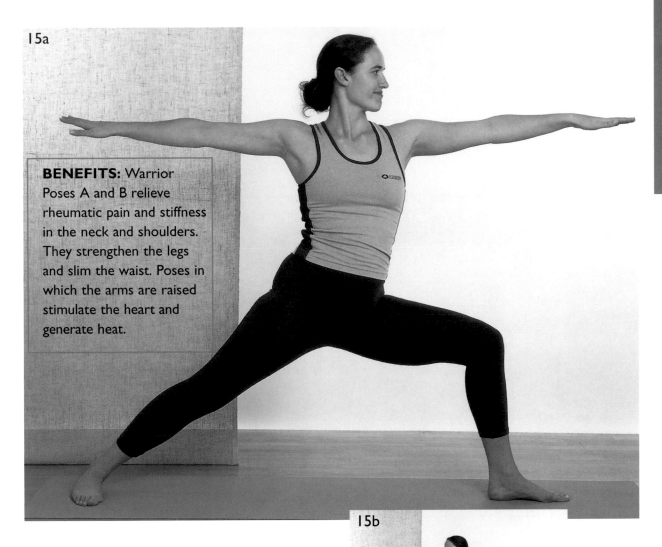

**BENEFITS:** Warrior Poses A and B relieve rheumatic pain and stiffness in the neck and shoulders. They strengthen the legs and slim the waist. Poses in which the arms are raised stimulate the heart and generate heat.

15b

## 15 Warrior Pose B

*Virabhadrasana B*
Start from the end position of Warrior Pose A.

**Exhale:** keep your left leg bent at 90°, and turn your hips, head, and torso to face forward. Lower your arms to shoulder height, with your left arm forward, your right arm back, and your palms facing the floor (see 15a). Look over your left shoulder, but keep the right side of your body pulling back, so that your torso remains centered over your pelvis and between your feet.

**Breath:** remain in this pose for five breaths.

**Inhale:** straighten the bent leg, turn your feet to the right side, and repeat the pose (see 15b).

**Exhale:** bend forward over the right leg and place your hands on either side of the right foot. Take the right foot back in line with the left foot. Lower into the Four-Limbed Stick (see p. 38).

**Inhale:** move into the Upward Dog (see p. 38).

**Exhale:** move into the Downward Dog (see p. 39).

**Inhale:** jump through the hands, straight into a sitting position, ready for the sitting poses (see p. 72).

# fast index to the standing poses

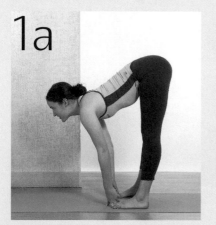

1a

Forward Bend A

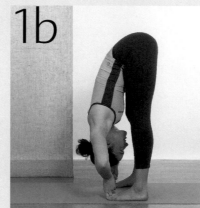

1b

Forward Bend A

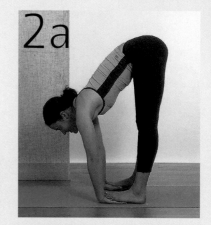

2a

Forward Bend B

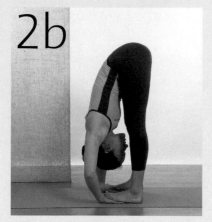

2b

Forward Bend B

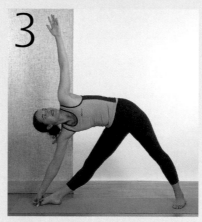

3

Extended Triangle

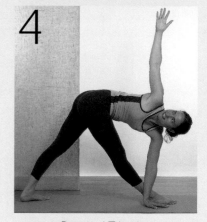

4

Reversed Triangle

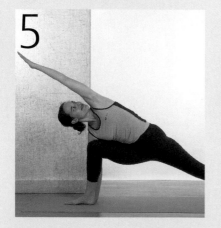

5

Extended Sideways Pose

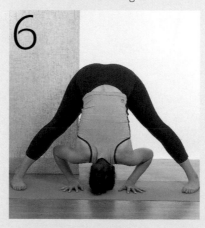

6

Spread-Leg Pose A

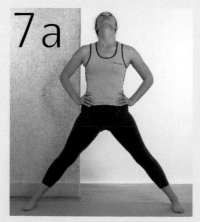

7a

Spread-Leg Pose B

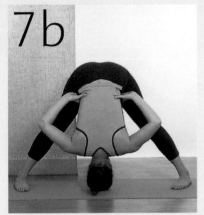

7b

Spread-Leg Pose B

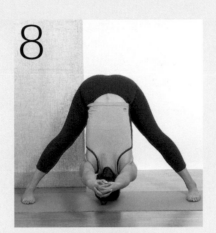

8

Spread-Leg Pose C

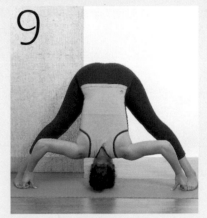

9

Spread-Leg Pose D

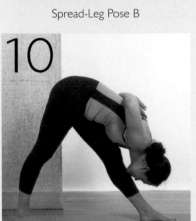

10

Sideways Extension

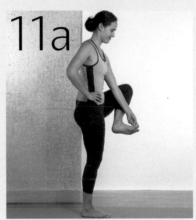

11a

Thumb-to-Foot Pose

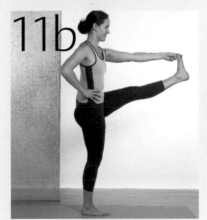

11b

Thumb-to-Foot Pose

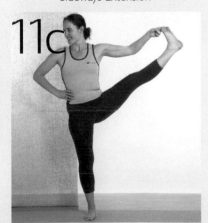

11c

Thumb-to-Foot Pose

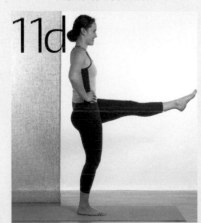

11d

Thumb-to-Foot Pose

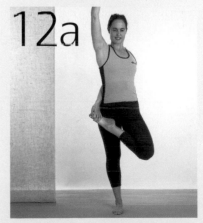

12a

Half-Bound Lotus Stretch

# fast index continued

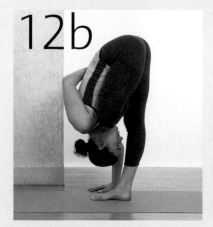

Half-Bound Lotus Stretch

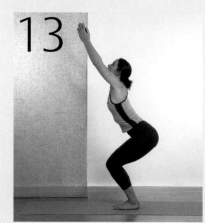

Uneven Pose

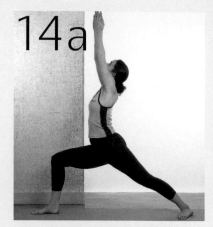

Warrior Pose A

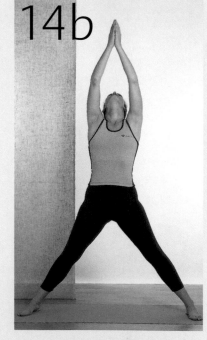

Warrior Pose A

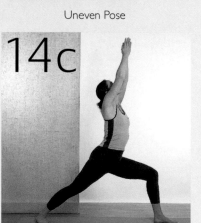

Warrior Pose A

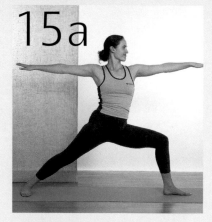

Warrior Pose B

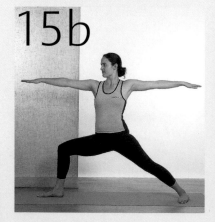

Warrior Pose B

## WARNING

■ Do not attempt either of the Warrior Poses if you have a heart condition of any sort.

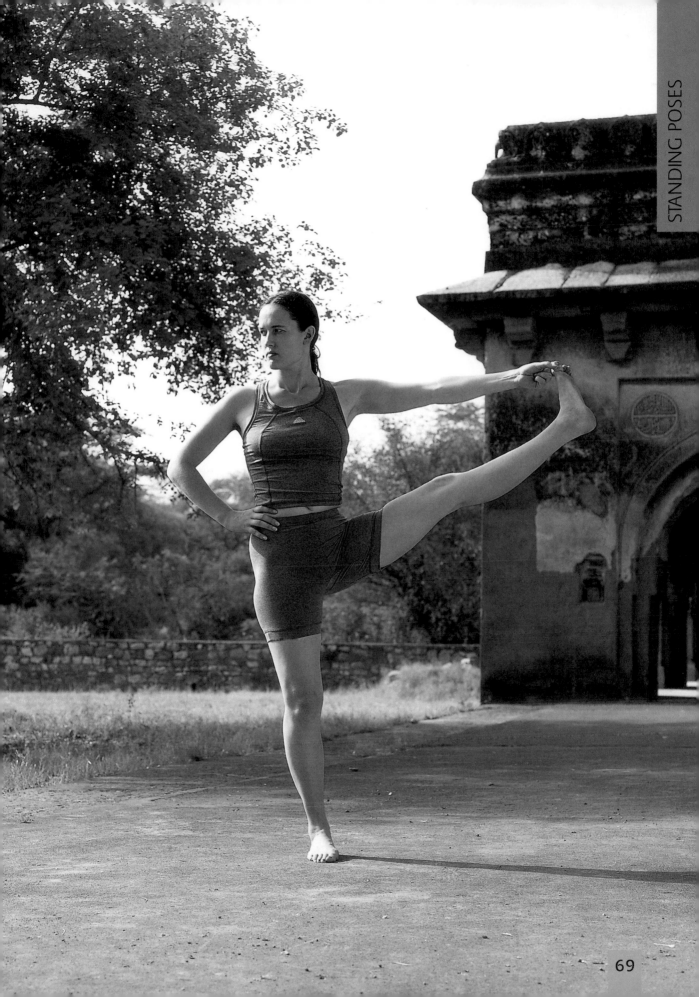

CHAPTER THREE

# Sitting poses

Sitting poses fall into two categories: forward bends, whereby the trunk bends over the legs; and spinal twists, in which the spine rotates to both left and right. The sitting poses calm the mind, bringing a fresh supply of oxygen to the brain, which aids restful sleep. They stretch the entire back, creating enhanced flexibility, and they relieve sciatic pains caused by compression in the spine and tone the spinal nerves. The forward bends strengthen and elongate the hamstrings. The sitting twists massage the abdominal organs and aid the digestive system. They also improve side-to-side flexibility in the spine, removing stiffness in the neck and shoulders.

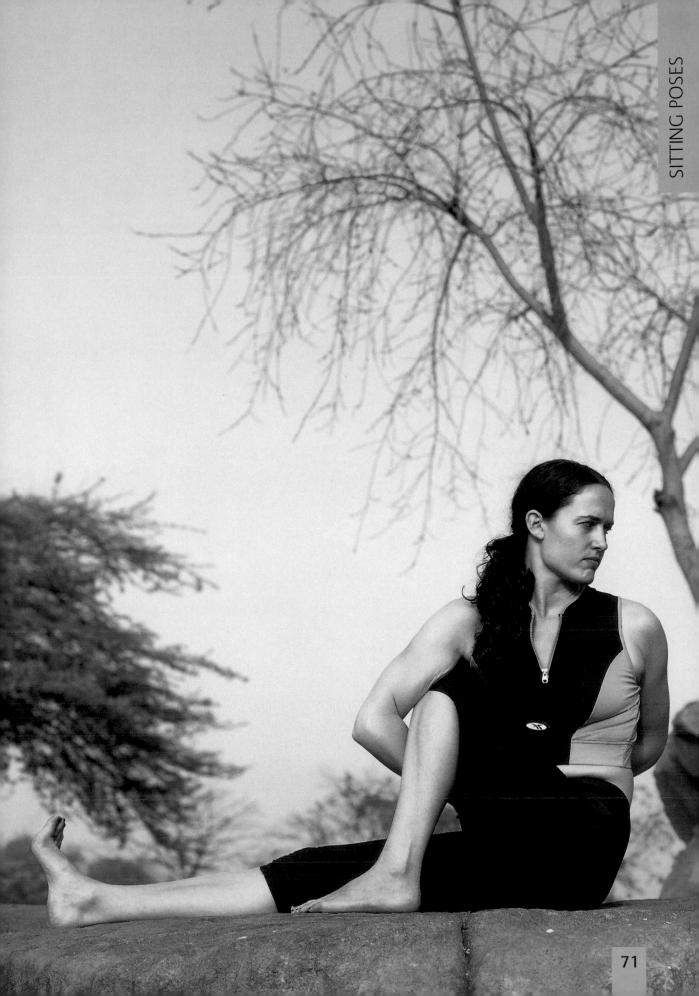

# Forward **bends**

*Do not skip any poses that you find difficult. With patience and diligent practice you will be able to master them, and then move on to the next pose in the sequence.*

**Sitting Extension**
*Dandasana*
**Exhale:** in a seated position, press your palms into the floor on either side of your buttocks, tightly draw in your stomach muscles, and apply mula bandha (see p. 25). Lift your chest and tuck your chin in. Keep your heels pushing away.
**Breath:** rest for five breaths.

## TECHNIQUE: THE HALF-VINYASA

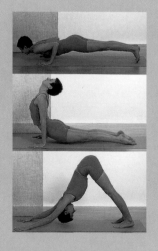

■ Vinyasa distinguishes Ashtanga yoga from other schools. It means "breath-synchronized movement". A Full Vinyasa refers to the Salute to the Sun A. In sitting postures, a Half-Vinyasa is practiced. Between each sitting pose, inhale and press both palms into the ground, then try to lift your trunk and legs off the floor. Either roll over your toes and spring back, or swing your raised body into the Four-Limbed Stick (see p. 38). As you inhale, roll over your toes into the Upward Dog (see p. 38). As you exhale, push into your palms and raise your buttocks, going into the Downward Dog (see p. 39). From here, inhale as you jump your feet through your hands, into the next sitting position.

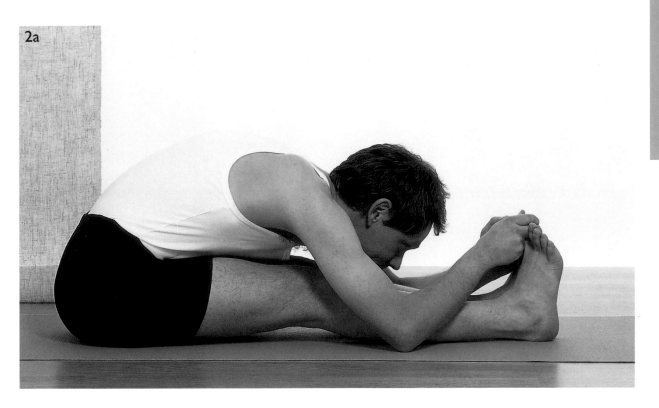

2a

## 2 Back Extension
*Paschimottanasa*

**Inhale:** lift your arms over your head and stretch up from the base of your spine.

**Exhale:** bend forward and catch hold of your big toes with the thumbs and forefingers of both hands, while keeping your legs straight. Bend your elbows out to the sides and take your head down between your legs (see 2a).

**Breath:** hold for five breaths.

**Inhale:** straighten your arms, lift your head, and stretch up along your spine.

**Exhale:** take hold of the sides of your feet and bend forward between your legs (see 2b).

**Breath:** hold for five breaths.

**Inhale:** straighten your arms again, lift your head, and stretch your spine.

**Exhale:** for a more advanced stretch, take hold of your left wrist with your right hand behind the soles of your feet, then take your head down to your legs (see 2c).

**Breath:** hold for five breaths.

**Inhale:** come up to a sitting position.

**Exhale:** lift your body up and do a Half-Vinyasa.

■ **Beginners:** if you cannot yet reach your feet, then reach as far down the leg as is possible and work from that position. The same applies to all the forward bends.

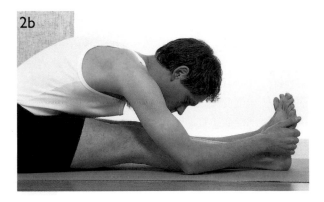

2b

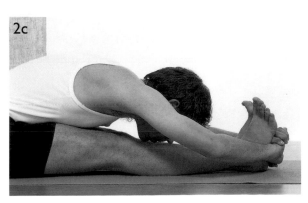

2c

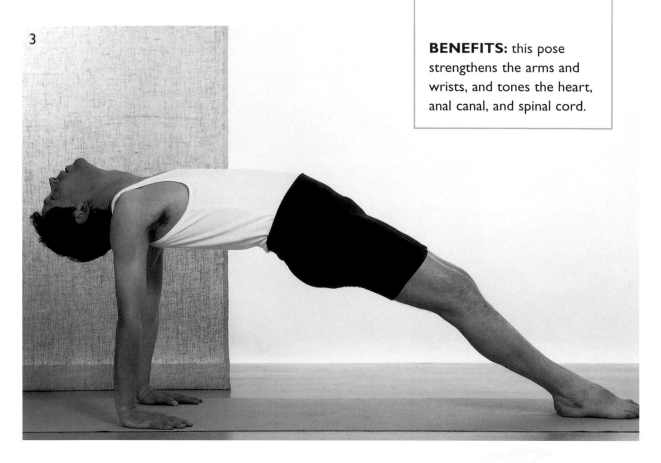

3

**BENEFITS:** this pose strengthens the arms and wrists, and tones the heart, anal canal, and spinal cord.

## 3 Forward Extension

*Purvottanasana*

This posture acts as a counterstretch to the previous series of forward bends. It stretches the entire front of the body, from the toes to the head.

**Inhale:** sit with your legs facing forward.

**Exhale:** place your hands behind your back, about 1 foot/30 cm from your buttocks, with your fingers facing forward. Point your toes away from your body toward the floor.

**Inhale:** on a deep inhalation, press into your palms and lift your chest and hips into the air. Put your big toes and feet flat on the floor and lean your head back.

**Breath:** hold your body tightly in this position for five breaths.

**Exhale:** lower your body back into a sitting position.

**Inhale:** lift your body up and do a Half-Vinyasa.

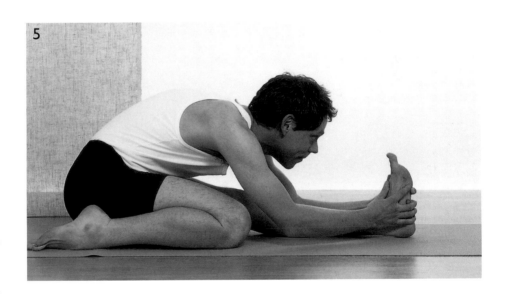

## 4 Half-Bound Foot
*Ardha Baddha Padma Paschimottanasana*

**Inhale:** sit with your legs facing forward. Bend your right leg and place its ankle on top of your left thigh. Rotate your right leg so that your knee touches the floor. To bind the leg, lift and stretch your right arm and take it around your back, grabbing hold of your right big toe. Keep your left leg pressing into the floor.

**Exhale:** bend forward over the extended leg and take hold of your left foot with your left hand. Place your head on your left leg.

**Breath:** remain in this position for a duration of five breaths.

**Inhale:** come up and release the foot.

**Exhale:** sit up straight.

**Inhale:** bend your left leg and repeat the pose on the left side. Do a Half-Vinyasa into the next position.

## 5 Three-Limbed Forward Bend
*Triang Mukhaikapada Paschimottanasana*

**Inhale:** come to a sitting position with legs facing forward. Bend your right leg back, moving the calf muscle out to the right. The right foot should point backward, with the heel up. Make sure that the center top of your right foot is resting on the floor. Sit up straight and try to distribute the weight of your body evenly on both buttock bones.

**Exhale:** raise your body up and bend forward over your extended left leg. Hold your left foot and take your chin down to the left leg. Try to keep both buttocks on the floor.

**Breath:** remain in this position for five breaths.

**Inhale:** come up to a sitting position.

**Exhale:** release the right leg and sit up straight, with both legs forward.

**Inhale:** bend the left leg.

**Exhale:** repeat the pose on the left side. Do a Half-Vinyasa into the next position.

6

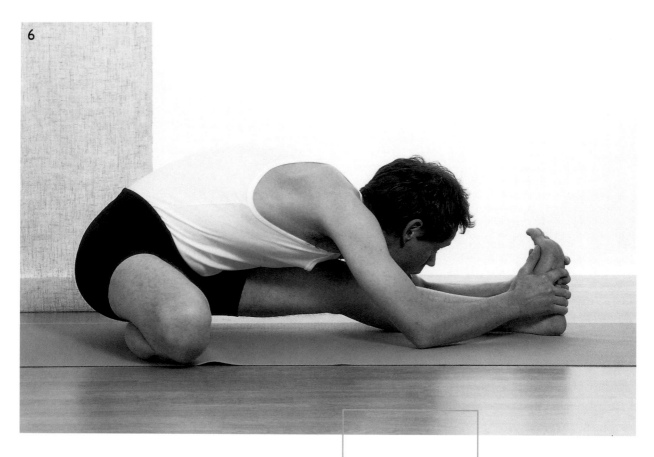

## 6 Head-to-Knee Pose A

*Janu Shirshasana A*
**Inhale:** from a seated position, bend your right leg and take the knee out to the side. Your right foot should press alongside your inner left thigh. Sit up and turn your body so that it is facing forward and toward the center of the left leg.
**Exhale:** bend forward and take hold of your left foot. Bend forward over your straight left leg, keeping both sides of the leg parallel. Take your chin down to your shin.
**Breath:** hold this position for five breaths.
**Inhale:** come up to a sitting position and straighten your right leg.
**Exhale:** sit up straight, or perform a Half-Vinyasa.
**Inhale:** bend your left leg and repeat the pose on the left side. Do a Half-Vinyasa into the next position.

**BENEFITS:** practicing this Ashtanga pose helps to improve flexibility in the spine, and it also lengthens the hamstrings.

## 7 Head-to-Knee Pose B

*Janu Shirshasana B*
**Inhale:** from a seated position, bend your right leg out to the side at an angle of 85°, with the sole of your right foot running along the inside of your left thigh. Press both hands into the floor on either side of your buttocks and lift your body up and forward, placing your anus directly on top of your right heel. Apply mula bandha and uddiyana bandha

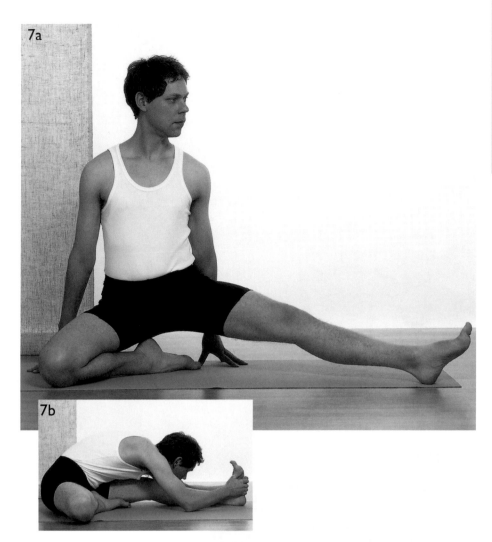

7a

7b

(see p. 25). Still sitting on top of your right heel, turn your body to face forward toward your left leg (see 7a).

**Exhale:** bend forward and take hold of your left foot. Take your chin down to your shin (see 7b).

**Breath:** hold this position for five breaths.

**Inhale:** come up and release the pose.

**Exhale:** sit up straight.

**Inhale:** bend your left leg out to the side and repeat the pose on the left side.

Do a Half-Vinyasa into the next position.

**8 Head-to-Knee Pose C** *Janu Shirshasana C*

**Inhale:** stretch your left leg forward. Bend and lift your right leg, turn the calf muscle toward you and twist the foot. Place your toes on the floor, so that your heel faces toward your navel. Apply mula bandha and uddiyana bandha (see p. 25).

**Exhale:** bend forward and take hold of your left foot with both hands, then bring your body down over your left leg, taking your chin down to your shin.

**Breath:** hold the position for five breaths.

**Inhale:** come up and release the right leg.

**Exhale**: sit up straight, or perform a Half-Vinyasa.

**Inhale:** bend the left leg and repeat the pose on the left side.

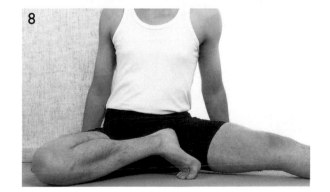

8

Do a Half-Vinyasa into the next position.

# Spinal twists & balances

*The twists gently massage the internal organs of the body, especially the intestines and the kidneys. Practice them in the order in which they are given here, for maximum benefit.*

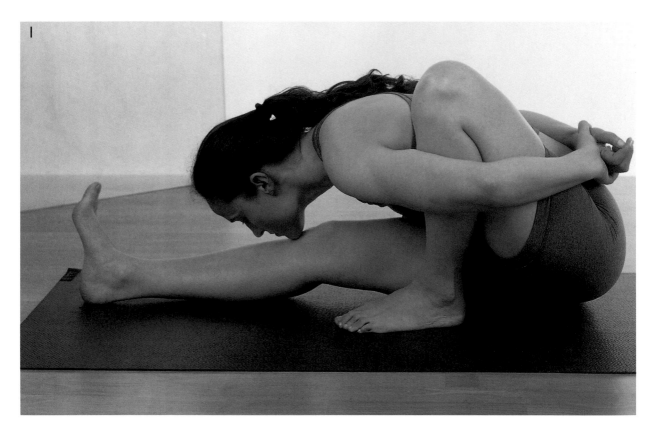

**Marici Pose A**
*Maricyasana A*
*Note that Marici Poses A, B, C, and D should begin on the right side, but they are shown here on the left side for variation.*
**Inhale:** sit straight with the legs forward. With the right leg strong, bend your left leg and place the heel as close to your inner thighs as possible. Extend your left arm inside your bent left leg toward your right foot, bending forward over your extended right leg. Then wrap your left arm around your bent leg and take your right arm behind your back. Clasp your right wrist with your left hand.

**Exhale:** take your chest closer to your right leg, with right leg straight and bent left leg vertical. Rest your chin on your shin.

**Breath:** hold for five long breaths.
**Inhale:** come up and relax your right leg.
**Exhale:** sit straight, or perform a Half-Vinyasa.
**Inhale:** repeat on the other side. Do a Half-Vinyasa into the next position.

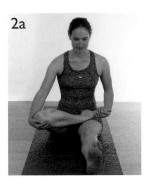

2a

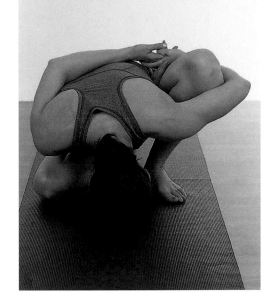

2b

## 2 Marici Pose B
### *Maricyasana B*

**Inhale:** bend your right leg and bring the foot to your left groin, cradling your knee (see 2a). Take the right knee toward the floor. Straighten your trunk by pressing into your fingertips. Bend your left knee and place the heel close to your left buttock.

**Exhale:** bend for-ward, inside your bent leg. Stretch your left arm forward and wrap it back around the left leg, taking your right arm behind your back and holding hands. Take your head to the floor (see 2b).

**Breath:** hold for five long breaths.

**Exhale:** move into a seated position, or perform a Half-Vinyasa.

**Inhale:** repeat on the other side. Then do a Half-Vinyasa into the next position.

## 3 Marici Pose C
### *Maricyasana C*

**Inhale:** bend your left leg, placing the heel close to your left buttock, with the right leg on the floor.

**Exhale**: rotate your upper body so it faces the bent left leg. Bend your right arm around the outside of the left knee. Take your left arm behind your back, grabbing your wrist. Look over the left shoulder.

**Breath:** hold for five long breaths.

**Exhale:** move into a seated position, or do a Half-Vinyasa.

**Inhale:** repeat on the other side. Do a Half-Vinyasa into the next position.

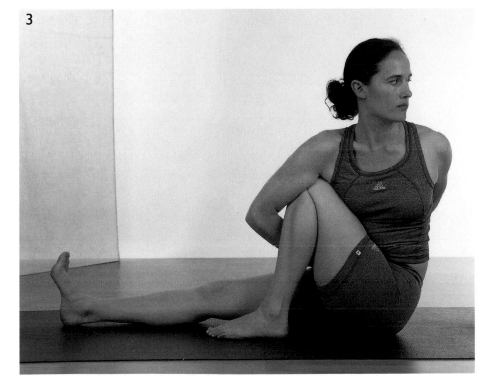

3

4b

4a

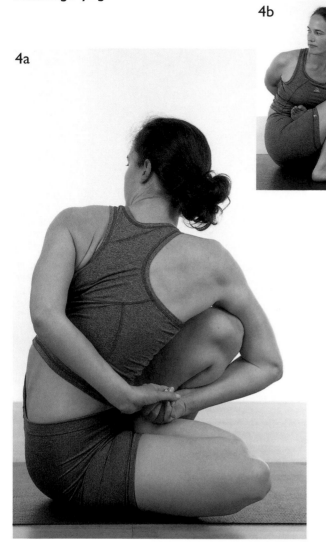

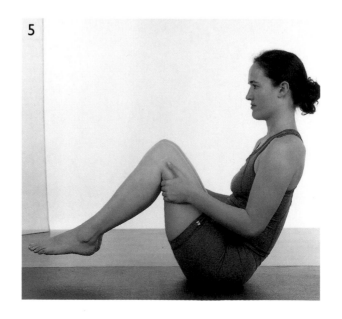

**4 Marici Pose D**
*Maricyasana D*
**Inhale:** sit straight and bend your right leg, placing your right foot into your left groin and bringing your left knee to the floor. Then bend your left leg, bringing the heel of the left foot close to your left buttock and assuming the same initial posture as in Marici Pose B.
**Exhale:** rotate your trunk toward the left leg and take your right upper arm around the outside of your left knee. Using your right arm as a lever, try to increase the rotation of your upper body. Wrap your right arm around the outside of your left leg, take your left arm behind your back and hold hands. Look over your left shoulder (see 4a.)
**Breath:** hold for five long breaths.
**Exhale:** sit straight with your legs together, or perform a Half-Vinyasa.
**Inhale:** repeat the pose on the other side (see 4b). Do a Half-Vinyasa into the next position.
**Beginners:** the poses that help prepare the body for Marici Poses B and D are the Half-Bound Lotus Stretch in the standing sequence (see p. 62) and the Half-Bound Foot earlier in the sitting sequence (see p. 74). Master them before attempting Marici Poses B and D.

5

**5 Boat Pose A**
*Navasana A*
**Inhale:** bend your knees and place your heels about 1½ feet/ 45 cm from your buttocks. Hold the backs of your knees with both hands and then gently roll backward until you are just balancing on your buttocks. Move into Boat Pose B.

## 6 Boat Pose B
### Navasana B

When balanced on the buttocks, straighten your legs. Keep your arms straight, with your hands facing each other at knee height. Your gaze should be along the plane of your nose.

**Breath:** hold for five breaths.

**Inhale:** place your hands on either side of your buttocks, bend your knees, and cross your legs, keeping your feet off the floor. Lift your body, using the strength of your arms.

**Exhale:** come back down and repeat the pose again.

**Breath:** hold for five breaths. Repeat the Boat series three to six times, with a lift between each pose.

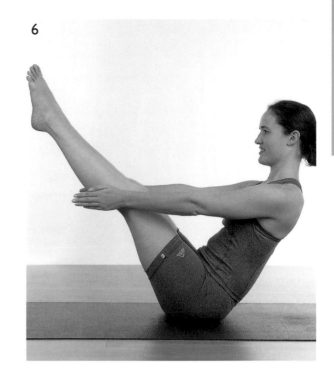

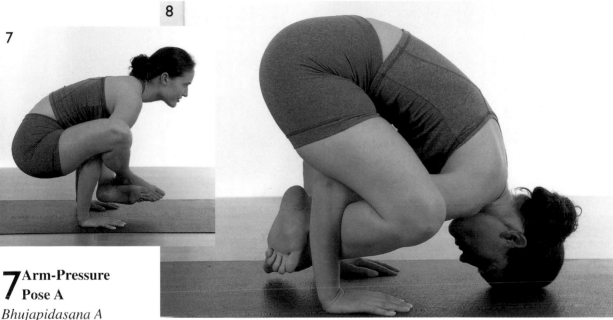

## 7 Arm-Pressure Pose A
### Bhujapidasana A

**Inhale:** from the Downward Dog (see p. 39), jump your feet to the outsides of your arms, just in front of your hands. Crouch, and bend your elbows backward, resting the backs of your thighs high on your upper arms. Balance on your hands; lift both feet. Cross your right foot over the left; straighten your arms. Look along the plane of your nose.

## 8 Arm-Pressure Pose B
### Bhujapidasana B

**Exhale:** bend your elbows backward, then rotate your body and take your crossed feet between your arms. Place your forehead on the floor.

**Breath:** hold for five breaths.

**Exhale:** lift your head, bring your feet forward, and straighten your legs.

# Advanced sitting poses

*Once you have mastered the forward bends and spinal twists, you can move on to these more advanced sitting poses, some of which require the assistance of a partner or teacher to help you achieve the correct position.*

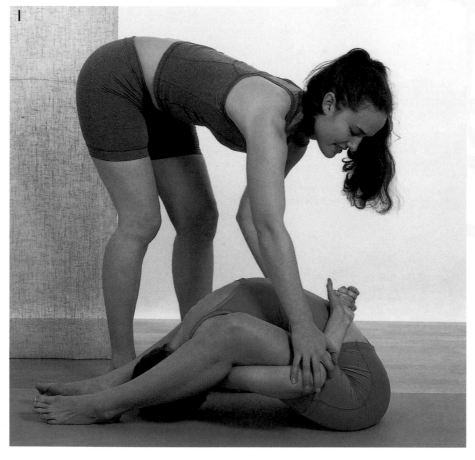

**Tortoise**
*Kurmasana*
**Inhale:** from the Downward Dog pose (see p. 39), jump your feet to the outside of your hands, so that you are in a squatting position. Then take your arms through your bent legs and lower your buttocks to the floor. Bend forward, taking your chin and chest to the floor, and straighten your arms out to the sides and slightly back. Then straighten your legs, which should be resting on your upper arms, close to your shoulders and pointing forward. Press your heels away from you and your toes toward you to give a complete stretch through the backs of your legs.

**Breath:** stay in this position with your head tucked under for five complete breaths.

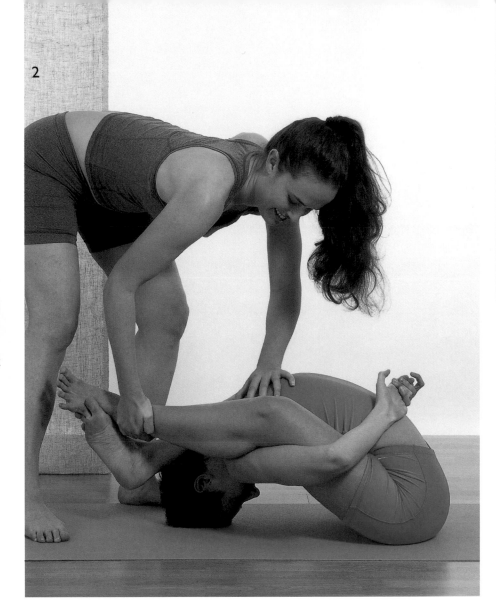

2

## 2 Sleeping Tortoise
*Supta Kurmasana*

**Caution:** if you are a beginner, the next part of the exercise should be attempted only with the help of a teacher.

**Exhale:** from the previous pose, your teacher will bring your hands behind your back so that you are able to take hold of your left wrist with your right hand. After you have placed your forehead on the floor, he or she will then lift your right leg and place your right foot behind your head, and will then lift your left leg and cross the left foot over the right foot.

**Breath:** take five full breaths.

**For advanced practitioners, and those who are working with the help of a teacher:** inhale and release your hands, and place them alongside your buttocks. Pressing into your palms, lift your head and torso, with your feet still crossed behind your head.

**Exhale:** steady the pose.

**Inhale:** lift your buttocks off the floor.

**Exhale:** release your feet, bend your knees, and place your feet on the outside of your hands.

**Inhale:** find your balance.

**Exhale:** jump back into the Four-Limbed Stick pose (see p. 38) for a Half-Vinyasa (see p. 72). More adept practitioners can bend their knees and, without touching their feet to the floor, remain balanced on their elbows and jump back from there.

**BENEFITS:** this pose purifies the area from which all the 72,000 nadi emanate, which is called the khanda (see p. 26). The spinal column is also strengthened. The senses are retracted from external stimuli.

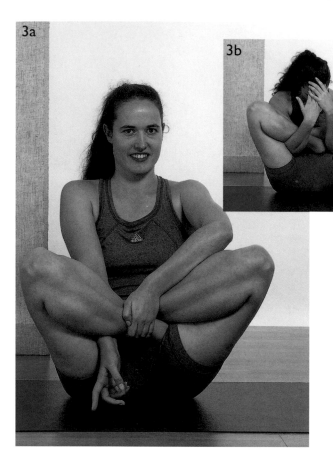

3a

3b

## 3 Embryo in the Womb

*Garbha Pindasana*

**Inhale:** Assume the Lotus Position *(Padmasana),* by bending your right leg and placing your right ankle on top of your left thigh; then bend your left leg and place your left ankle on top of your right thigh. Lift your crossed legs and, holding your right knee with your left hand, push your right arm through the bend of the right leg, between the thigh and calf (see 3a). If you have a lot of perspiration, your arm should slip though easily, past the elbow. Then push your left arm through the bend in your left leg, while balancing on your buttocks. Hold the side of your head close to your ears with both hands.

**Breath:** hold for five breaths.

**Inhale:** bend your head forward, taking your chin toward your breastbone, and hold your head with both hands (see 3b).

**Exhale:** keeping your spine rounded, rock backward and forward nine times (see 3c). After each full roll, shift clockwise and roll again, so that after nine rolls you are facing the original direction.

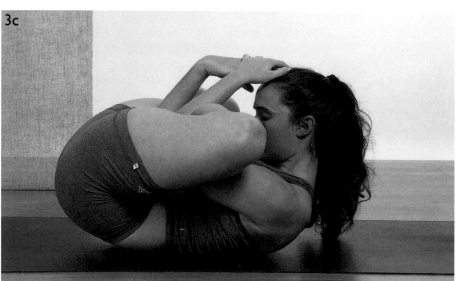

3c

**BENEFITS:** this asana strengthens the uterus. It tones and cleanses the liver and spleen and purifies the manipura-chakra (see p. 28).

## 4 Rooster Pose
*Kukkutasana*

**Inhale:** on the last forward roll of Step 3c, propel yourself upright onto your hands, palms pressing into the floor, so you are balancing on your arms with your buttocks and legs raised off the floor. Lift your back and chest fully. Apply uddiyana bandha (see p. 25), but release mula bandha (see p. 25).

**Breath:** hold for five deep breaths.
**Exhale:** lower your buttocks and release your arms.
**Beginners**: unlock your legs, then swing back into the Four-Limbed Stick (see p. 38) for a Half-Vinyasa (see p. 72). Embryo in the Womb and the Rooster Pose take practice to master. First work on attaining the Lotus Position until you can main-

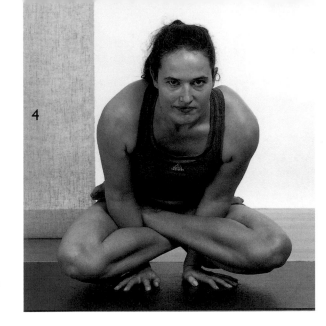

4

tain this comfortably; then proceed to the advanced stages.
**Advanced:** remain in the Lotus Position

and release your legs when you swing back into the Four-Limbed Stick pose.

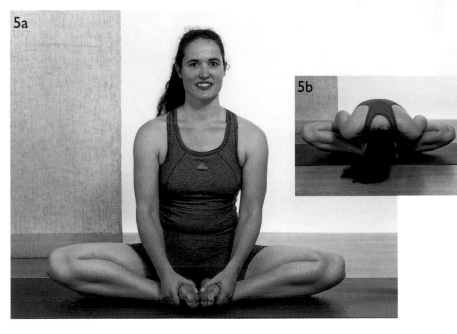

5a

5b

## 5 Bound Angle Pose
*Baddha Konasana*

**Inhale:** jump to a sitting position. Bend your knees and join the soles of your feet. Drop your knees out

to the sides and allow your soles to face upward. Hold your feet with your hands and try to take your knees to the floor. Lift your chest and tuck your chin in (see 5a).

**Exhale:** bend over your feet and take your chin to the floor (see 5b). Apply strong mula and uddiyana bandha (see p. 25).
**Breath:** hold for five breaths.

**Inhale:** come up and tuck your chin in.
**Exhale:** roll your spine into a ball and take the top of your head to your feet.
**Inhale:** come up and hold for five breaths.
**Exhale:** release the pose and bring your knees together.
**Inhale:** place your palms by your sides, with your fingers facing forward, and lift your body up.
**Exhale:** swing your legs backward for a Half-Vinyasa (see p. 72).

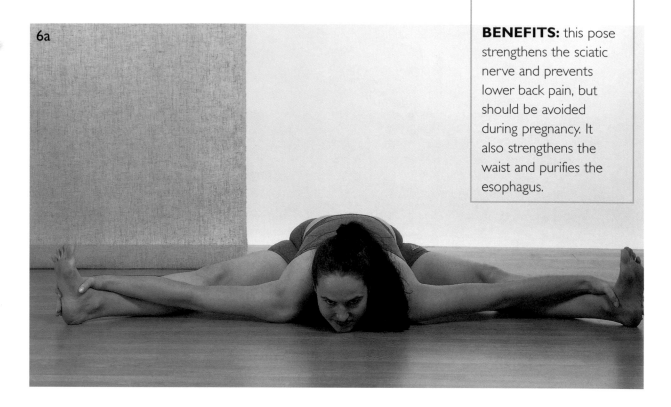

**BENEFITS:** this pose strengthens the sciatic nerve and prevents lower back pain, but should be avoided during pregnancy. It also strengthens the waist and purifies the esophagus.

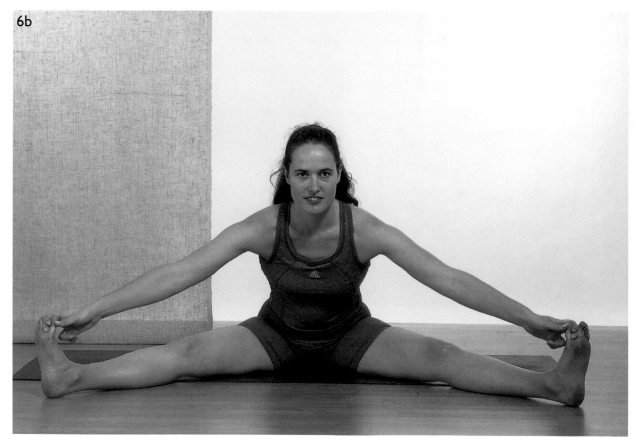

6c

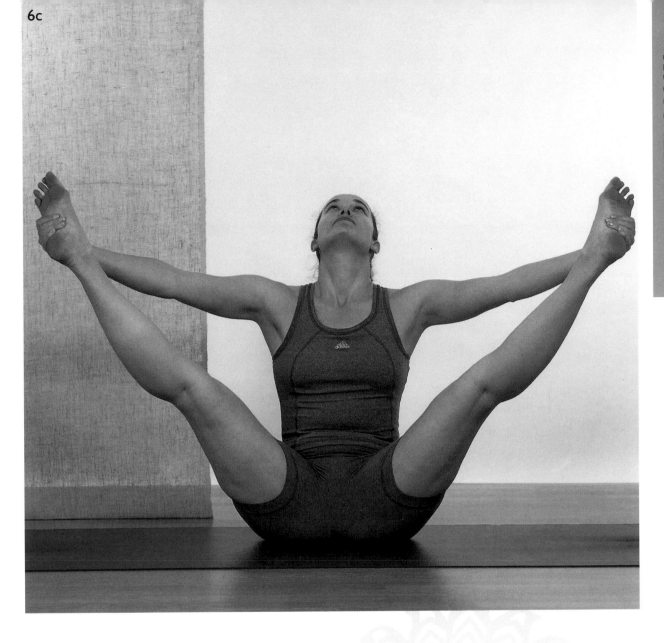

# 6 Seated Angle Pose

*Upavishta Konasana*

**Inhale:** jump to a sitting position and spread your legs as wide as possible. Take hold of the sides of both feet with your hands, lift your head and chest, and extend along your spine.

**Exhale:** draw in your stomach muscles and bend forward. Aim to place your chin and chest on the floor (see 6a).

**Breath:** hold for five breaths.

**Inhale:** lift your head and straighten your arms, while keeping hold of your feet (see 6b).

**Exhale:** in one movement pull your feet up until you are balancing solely on your buttock bones. Lift your head and look up toward the "third eye." Straighten your arms and the backs of your legs (see 6c). Apply both uddiyana and mula bandha (see p. 25).

**Breath:** hold for five breaths.

**Exhale:** release your feet and cross your legs in front of you. Place your palms down by your sides.

**Inhale:** lift up and swing your legs backward into the Four-Limbed Stick (see p. 38) for a Half-Vinyasa (see p. 72).

**Beginners:** it is very difficult to pull your legs up into the air in one movement, so initially you can bend your knees and balance on your buttocks, then straighten your legs.

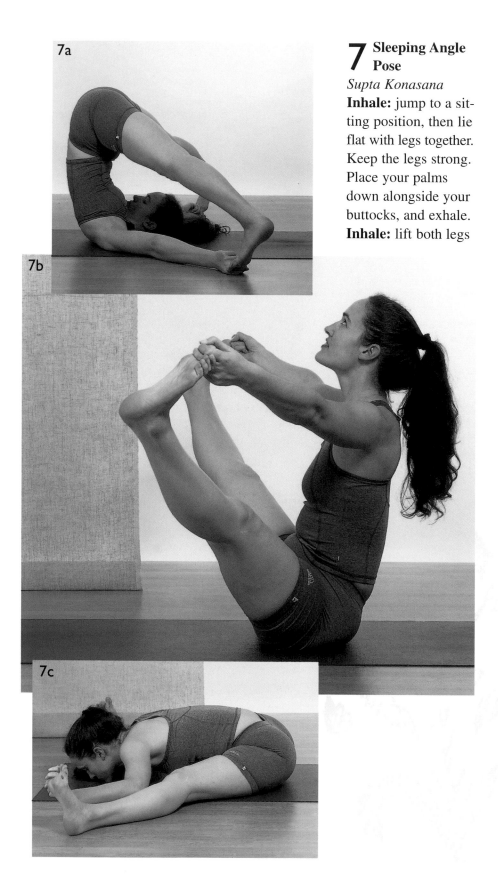

7a

7b

7c

## 7 Sleeping Angle Pose

*Supta Konasana*

**Inhale:** jump to a sitting position, then lie flat with legs together. Keep the legs strong. Place your palms down alongside your buttocks, and exhale.

**Inhale:** lift both legs up into an angle of 90° and press down into your palms.

**Exhale:** take your feet over your head and onto the floor behind you, spreading your legs as wide as possible and taking hold of your big toes (see 7a).

**Breath:** hold for five breaths.

**Inhale:** in one movement roll up into the Seated Angle Pose with your legs raised, while balancing on your buttock bones. Pull your stomach in, straighten your back, and look up (see 7b).

**Exhale:** lean forward and slowly roll down so that your legs are touching the floor. Bend forward, taking your chin and chest to the floor (see 7c).

**Inhale:** raise your head and straighten your arms, keeping hold of your feet.

**Exhale:** release your feet.

**Inhale:** sit up, cross your legs, and place your palms by your sides, then push up.

**Exhale:** swing your legs back into the Four-Limbed Stick (see p. 38) for a Half-Vinyasa (see p. 72).

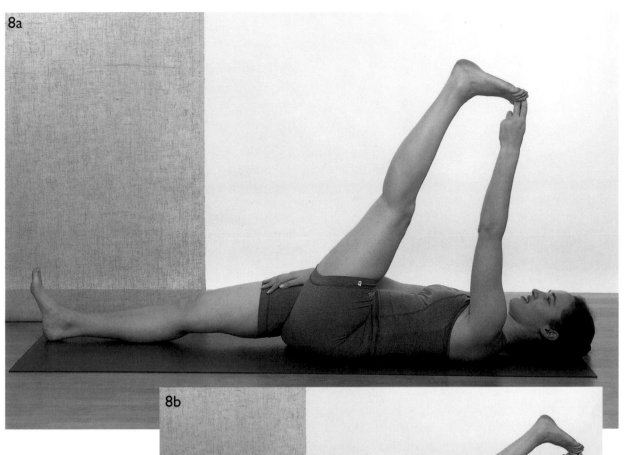

**8 Sleeping Thumb-to-Foot Pose** *Supta Padanghushtasana Note that this pose should begin on the right side, but is shown here on the left side for variation.*

**Inhale:** jump to a sitting position, then lie down with your legs together and your hands, palms down, by your sides. Keep your legs strong and exhale.

**Inhale:** with your right leg on the floor, lift your left leg to an angle of 90°. Hold of the left toe with your left hand and place your right hand on top of your right thigh to keep the leg pressed to the floor (see 8a).

**Exhale:** pull your left leg toward you and lift your head to touch your nose to your left knee (see 8b).

**Breath:** hold for five breaths.

**Inhale:** lower your head to the floor.

**Exhale:** lower your left leg back down to the floor.

**Inhale:** repeat the movement on the other side.

**Beginners:** doing a Half-Vinyasa between this pose and the next is optional.

**Advanced:** after finishing this pose, do a backward roll into the Four-Limbed Stick (see p. 38) by taking both feet up and over your head, rounding your spine, with hands directly underneath your shoulders, and elbows pointing up; push over and back.

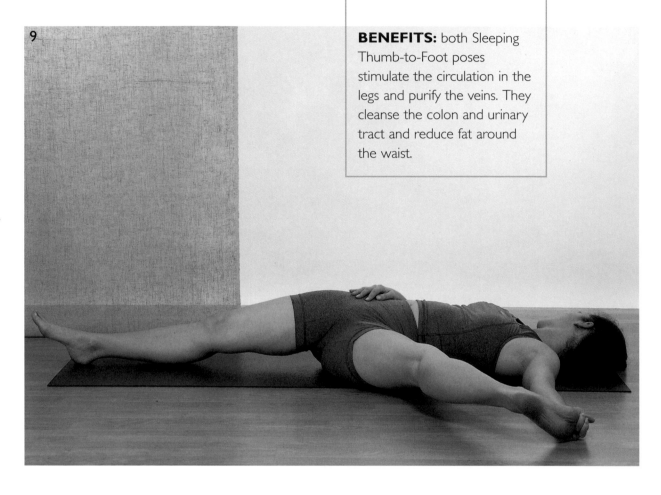

9

**BENEFITS:** both Sleeping Thumb-to-Foot poses stimulate the circulation in the legs and purify the veins. They cleanse the colon and urinary tract and reduce fat around the waist.

## 9 Lateral Sleeping Thumb-to-Foot Pose

*Supta Parsvasahita
Note that this pose should begin on the right side, but is shown here on the left side for variation.*
Repeat the two stages of the previous position (see p. 89).
**Inhale:** lower your head to the floor.
**Exhale:** lower your left leg out to the left side, while keeping hold of the big toe. Turn your head to look over your right shoulder.
**Breath:** hold this position for five breaths.
**Inhale:** bring your leg back to the center.
**Exhale:** pull your left leg toward you, then lift your head to touch your nose to the left knee.
**Inhale:** lower your head.
**Exhale:** lower your left leg back to the floor.
**Inhale:** repeat on the other side.

**Beginners:** perform vinyasa – on an inhalation, sit up, cross your legs, and place your palms down by your sides, then push up. Exhale and swing your legs back into the Four-Limbed Stick (see p. 38) for a Half-Vinyasa (see p. 72).
**Advanced:** do a backward roll (as above) into the Four-Limbed Stick for a Half-Vinyasa.

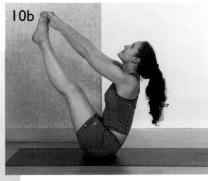

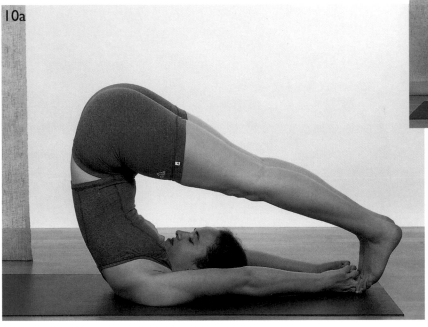

**WARNING:** if you are suffering from whiplash or neck problems, take medical advice before practicing this and the following two asanas.

**10 Both Thumbs-to-Feet Pose** *Ubhaya Padangusthasana*
**Inhale:** jump to a sitting position.
**Exhale:** lie down with your feet together and your arms alongside your body, with your palms on the floor.
**Inhale:** press into both palms and raise your legs up and over your body, then touch your toes to the floor behind your head, with the feet together. Hold both big toes with your thumbs and index fingers (see 10a).
**Exhale:** stay in this position for the duration of an exhalation.

**Inhale:** without letting go of your toes, roll forward until you are resting solely on your buttock bones. Your arms should be straight, your chest raised, and stomach muscles drawn. Lift your head up and back; look toward the "third eye" (see 10b).
**Breath:** hold for five complete breaths.
**Exhale:** let go of your toes and bring your hands, palms down, beside your buttocks.
**Inhale:** lift up your body.
**Exhale:** swing your legs back into the Four-Limbed Stick (see p. 38) for a Half-Vinyasa (see p. 72).

**11 Upward Forward Bend** *Urdhva Mukha Paschimattanasana*
**Inhale:** jump to a sitting position.
**Exhale:** lie down with legs together and

hands by your sides.
**Inhale:** as in the previous pose, lift your legs up and over your body, then place your toes on the floor behind your head (see 11a). Take hold of the

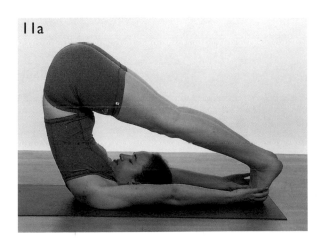

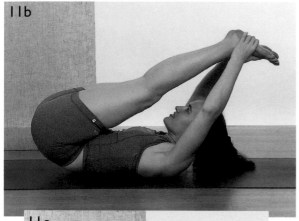

11b

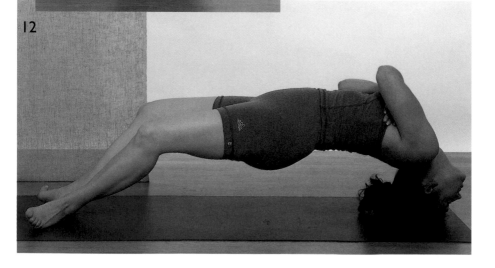

11c

sides of your feet, close to the heels (see 11b).

**Exhale:** hold and exhale.

**Inhale:** in one movement, roll forward until you are balancing solely on your buttock bones, still gripping both feet.

**Exhale:** bring your legs toward you, placing your head between your knees (see 11c).

**Breath:** take five slow breaths.

**Exhale:** straighten your legs, let go of your feet, and bring your hands, palms down, beside your buttocks.

**Inhale:** lift your body up.

**Exhale:** swing your legs back into the Four-Limbed Stick (see p. 38) for a Half-Vinyasa (see p. 72).

## 12 Bridge Pose
*Setu Bandhasana*

**Inhale:** jump to a sitting position.

**Exhale:** lie down with the feet together.

**Inhale:** remain in this position for the duration of an inhalation.

**Exhale:** bend your knees a little, turn your feet out at an angle of 45°, and bring your heels together, with the sides of your feet touching the floor. Bend back and place the top of your head on the floor. Straighten your legs and lift your chest, tucking your tailbone in and lifting your pubic bone.

**Inhale:** cross your arms over your chest so that you are balancing solely on your head and feet. Push through your heels and straighten legs.

**Exhale:** lower your body back to the floor.

12

*The following section is an advanced back-bending sequence.*

## 13 Upward Bow Pose

*Urdhva Dhanurasana*

**Inhale:** jump to a sitting position, then lie down.

**Exhale:** bend both knees and bring your heels close to your buttocks. Your feet should be hip-width apart and remain parallel. Bend your elbows and place your hands directly under your shoulders, with your fingers facing toward your feet. Tuck your tailbone in and move your pubic bone toward your head.

**Inhale:** remain in this position for the duration of an inhalation.

**Exhale:** pushing into both your palms and feet, lift your body up, raising your chest and pubic bone. Keep your legs and thighs strong and straighten through your elbows. Drop your head and look toward the tip of your nose.

**Beginners:** do an intermediate step by exhaling and lifting your body, resting the crown of your head on the floor; take two breaths, then push up into the full pose.

**Breath:** remain in this position for five breaths.

**Exhale:** gently lower your body back to the floor.

**Breath:** rest for a few moments, then repeat the pose three more times.

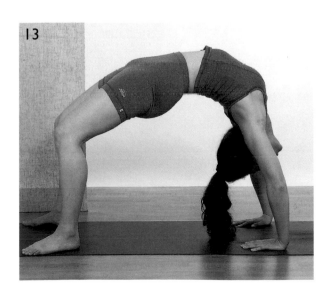

13

## 14 Working with a Partner in the Upward Bow Pose A

Stand with your feet hip-width apart and parallel. Cross your arms and tuck your hands under your armpits. Tuck your tailbone in. Your partner will hold you around the waist.

**Inhale:** stand tall and tuck your chin in.

**Exhale:** push forward into your pelvis to take your weight onto your thighs and toes. Bend backward as your partner holds you (see 14a).

**Inhale:** roll forward, then repeat the back-ward-and-forward roll in time with your breathing five times.

**Exhale:** roll back as far as possible. Then let your partner lower you until your head touches the floor (see 14b).

**Breath:** hold for five breaths.

**Inhale:** take one deep breath in as your partner lifts you to a standing position.

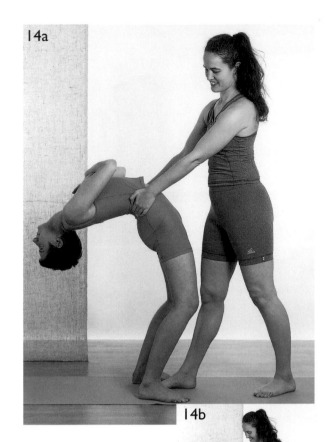

14a

14b

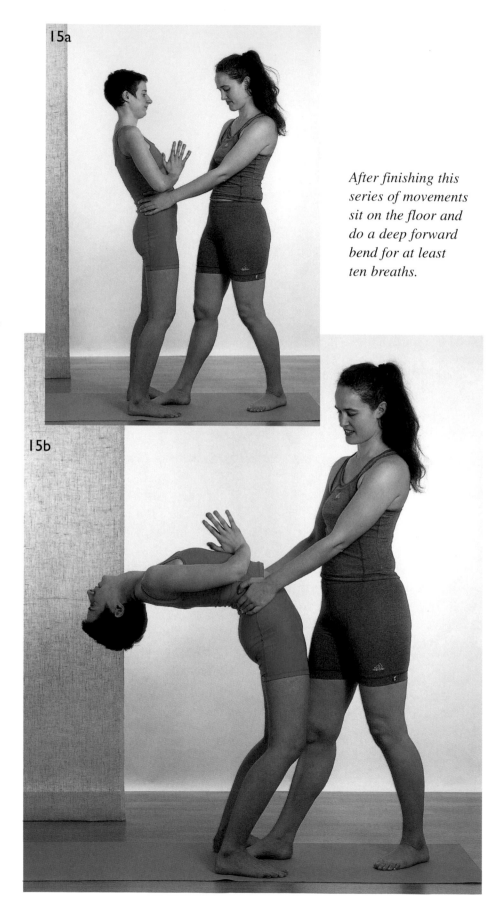

15a

15b

## 15 Working with a Partner in the Upward Bow Pose B

Stand with your feet hip-width apart and parallel. Cross your arms over your chest and tuck your hands under your armpits, or put them in the Prayer Position at waist level. Tuck your tail-bone in and extend through your spine. Your partner will hold you around the top of your hips (see 15a).
**Inhale:** stand tall.
**Exhale:** while your partner holds you, drop back and take your hands over your head, placing your palms on the floor (see 15b and 15c).
**Inhale:** push up as high as possible and try to walk your hands slightly closer to your heels (see 15d).
**Breath:** hold for five slow breaths.
**Exhale:** rock backward into your palms.
**Inhale:** in one movement rock forward and straighten up with the help of your partner.

*After finishing this series of movements sit on the floor and do a deep forward bend for at least ten breaths.*

94

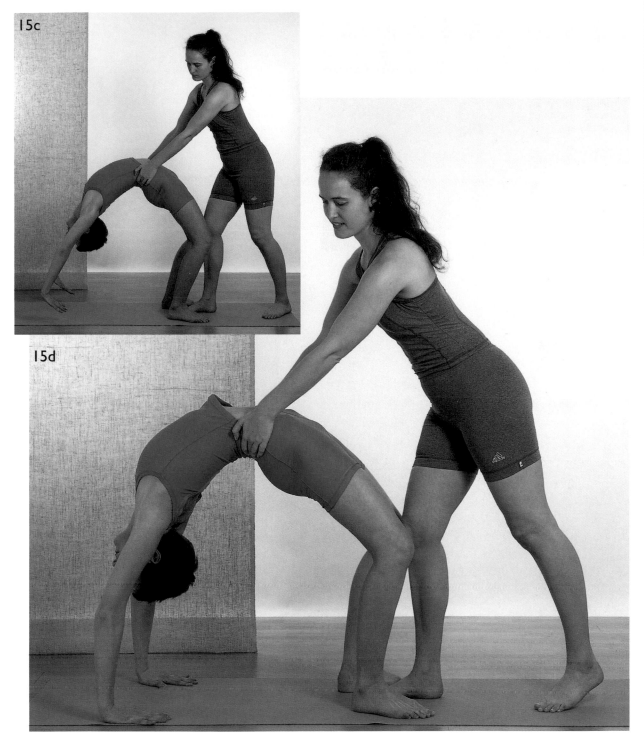

15c

15d

# BACK-BENDING

■ Back-bending helps to keep the spine strong and supple and prepares the

body for the more advanced poses in the second series. Always finish with a

Back Extension (see p. 73) to remove any knots in the spine.

# fast index to forward bends

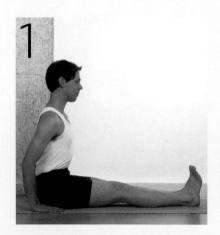

1

Sitting Extension

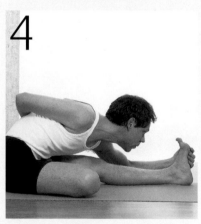

2a

Back Extension

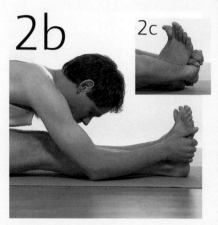

2b 2c

Back Extension

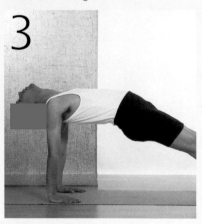

3

Forward Extension

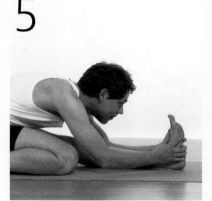

4

Half-Bound Foot

5

Three-Limbed Forward Bend

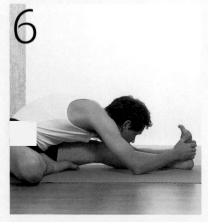

6

Head-to-Knee Pose A

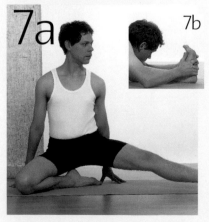

7a 7b

Head-to-Knee Pose B

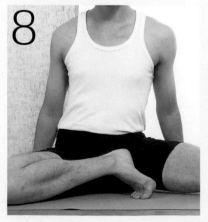

8

Head-to-Knee Pose C

# fast index to spinal twists & balances

**1**

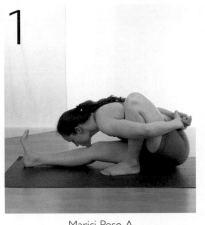

Marici Pose A

**2a**

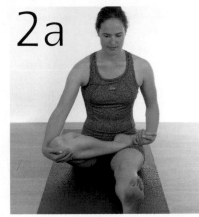

Marici Pose B

**2b**

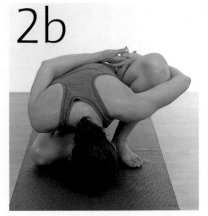

Marici Pose B

**3**

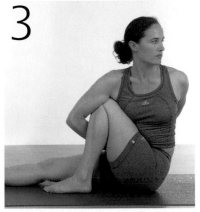

Marici Pose C

**4a** **4b**

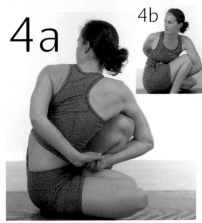

Marici Pose D

**5**

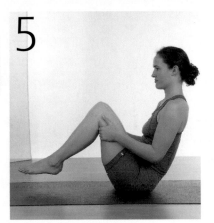

Boat Pose A

**6**

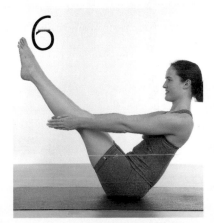

Boat Pose B

**7**

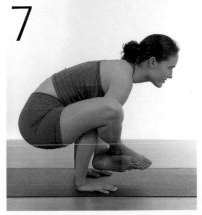

Arm-Pressure Pose A

**8**

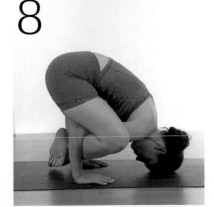

Arm-Pressure Pose B

# fast index to advanced sitting poses

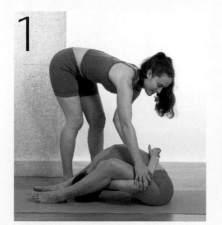
**1**

Tortoise

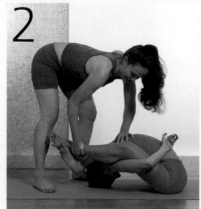
**2**

Sleeping Tortoise

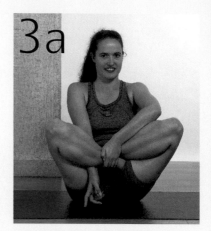
**3a**

Embryo in the Womb

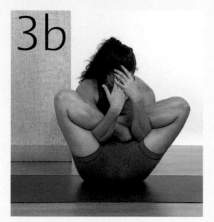
**3b**

Embryo in the Womb

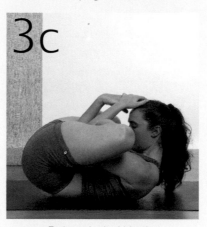
**3c**

Embryo in the Womb

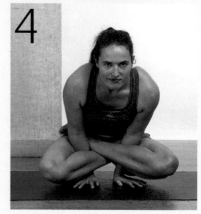
**4**

Rooster Pose

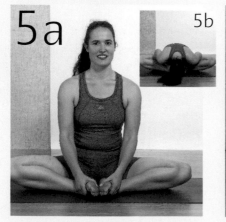
**5a** **5b**

Bound Ankle Pose

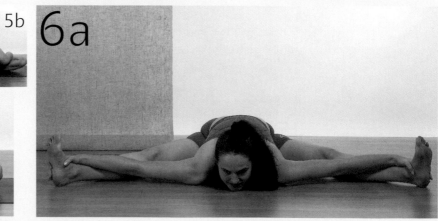
**6a**

Seated Angle Pose

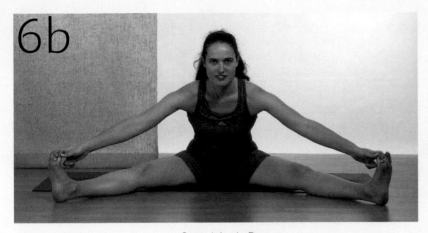

Seated Angle Pose

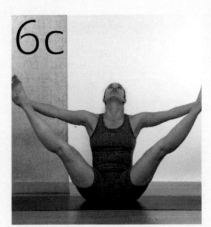

Seated Angle Pose

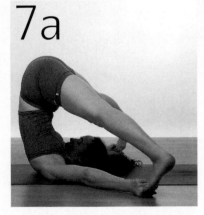

Sleeping Angle Pose

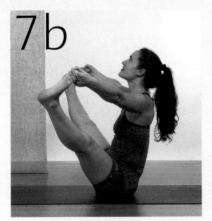

Sleeping Angle Pose

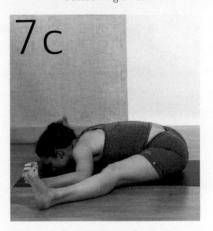

Sleeping Angle Pose

# BENEFITS OF WORKING WITH A PARTNER

■ In many of the more advanced Ashtanga poses it is very useful to work with another person, preferably your teacher or a fellow practitioner – someone who is familiar with the poses. To have support in the more difficult poses, like back-bending, builds your confidence until eventually you are able to drop back on your own.

# fast index to advanced sitting poses

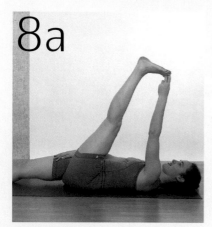

**8a**

Sleeping Thumb-to-Foot Pose

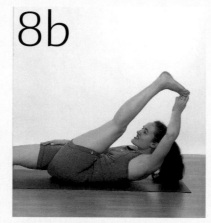

**8b**

Sleeping Thumb-to-Foot Pose

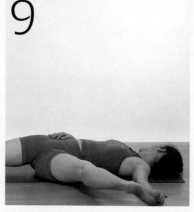

**9**

Lateral Sleeping Thumb-to-Foot Pose

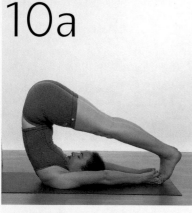

**10a**

Both Thumbs-to-Feet Pose

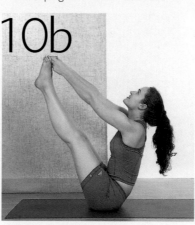

**10b**

Both Thumbs-to-Feet Pose

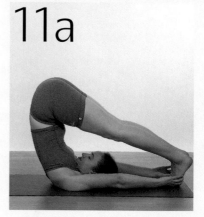

**11a**

Upward Forward Bend

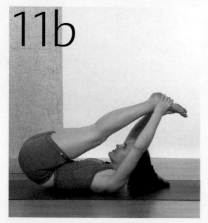

**11b**

Upward Forward Bend

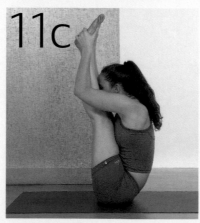

**11c**

Upward Forward Bend

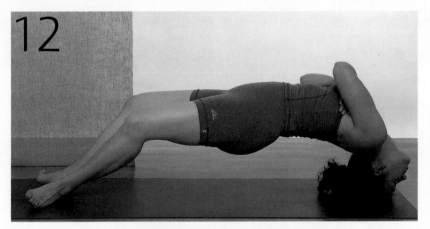
**12** Bridge Pose

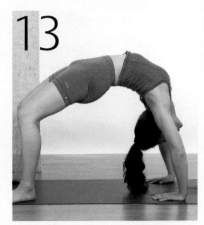
**13** Upward Bow Pose

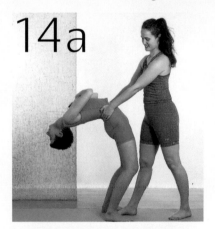
**14a** With a partner Upward Bow A

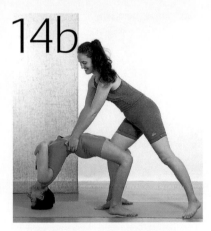
**14b** With a partner Upward Bow A

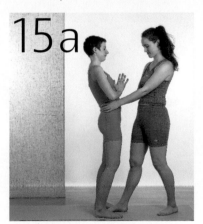
**15a** With a partner Upward Bow

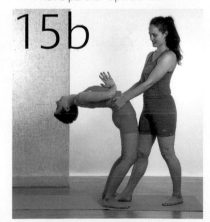
**15b** With a partner Upward Bow B

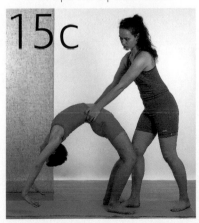
**15c** With a partner Upward Bow B

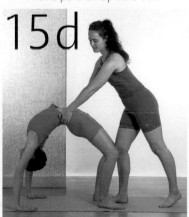
**15d** With a partner Upward Bow B

CHAPTER FOUR

# Finishing poses

There are two parts to the finishing sequence, both of which include an important inverted (upside-down) pose. The first part is a sequence of seven asanas, the first five of which form part of the All Limbs cycle, while the last two asanas are counterposes. Even if you do not complete all the poses in the primary series, always finish with the All Limbs cycle and then the Relax Pose (see p. 31). Beginners should learn these asanas in conjunction with the rest of the series. The second part emphasizes the Headstand Pose. This cycle is more difficult to master, and should be practiced by beginners only after the All Limbs cycle has been mastered.

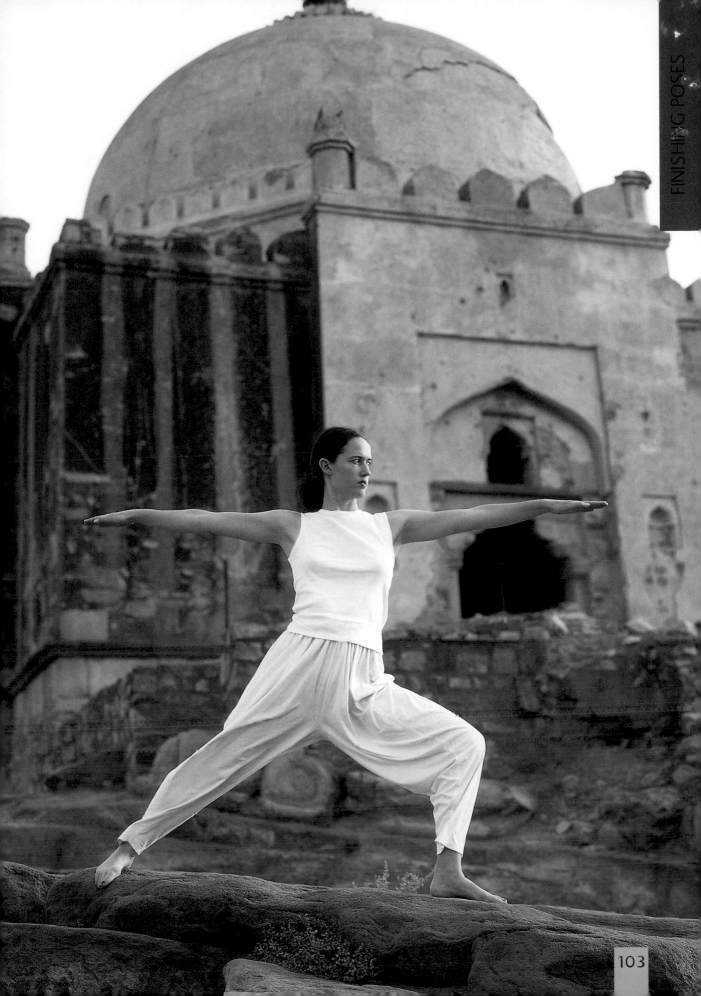

# All Limbs cycle

*This is so called because the entire body benefits from these poses. According to ancient yoga texts, the All Limbs Pose is the "queen" of asanas and of great importance, restoring harmony to the body after the practice of other poses.*

**WARNING:** do not practice this cycle if you are suffering from high blood pressure.

**All Limbs Pose**
*Salamba Sarvangasana*
**Inhale**: after a Half-Vinyasa jump through to a sitting position.
**Exhale:** lie down with your feet together and your arms by your sides.
**Breath:** rest in this position for five long breaths.
**Inhale:** tighten your knees and, by pressing into your palms, lift both legs up and over your head. At the same time lift your torso until your trunk is vertical and your chin is touching your breastbone, with your legs parallel to the floor. Stretch your arms away from your legs, then bend your elbows and support your hands on your back as far down toward the shoulders as possible. Lift your legs straight up into the air until your body is balanced on your shoulders, head, and neck. Look toward the tip of your nose. Keep the muscles in your

legs active and point your toes away from your head.

**Breath:** this pose can be held for up to half an hour; beginners are, however, advised to remain in this pose for just 25 breaths. You can do a backward roll into a Half-Vinyasa between each pose in the cycle, but as this would take a long time most practitioners move directly from one pose to the next.

**Beginners:** you can come up into this pose by bending both knees to your chest, then raising your hips off the floor and supporting them with your hands; gradually raise your trunk, supported by your hands, until your chin touches your chest. Finally straighten your legs.

**BENEFITS:** this asana cleanses the intestines and strengthens the waist and throat.

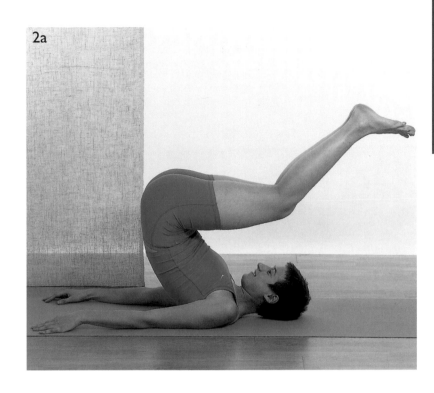

2a

## 2 Plow Pose
*Halasana*

**Exhale:** keeping your knees tightly together, lower your legs to the floor behind your head (see 2a). Place the tops of your feet on the floor, release your arms and stretch your hands away from your body, resting them on the floor. Your hips should be directly over your shoulders, with your chin tucked into your chest. Support your back with your hands (see 2b).

**Breath:** hold for 25 breaths.

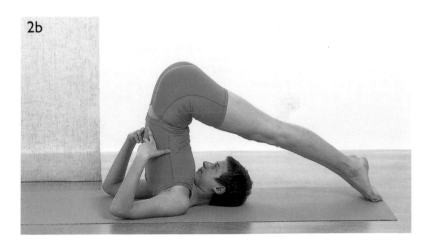

2b

3

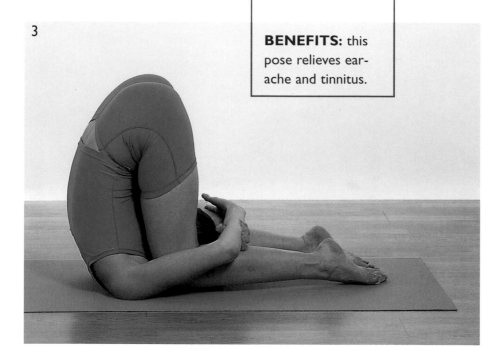

BENEFITS: this pose relieves ear-ache and tinnitus.

## 3 Ear-Pressure Pose

*Karnapidasana*

**Exhale:** bend both knees to the floor beside your ears and squeeze your ears with your knees. Wrap your arms over the tops of your calves. Relax mula bandha and apply uddiyana bandha (see p. 25).

**Breath:** remain in this position for 10 breaths.

4a

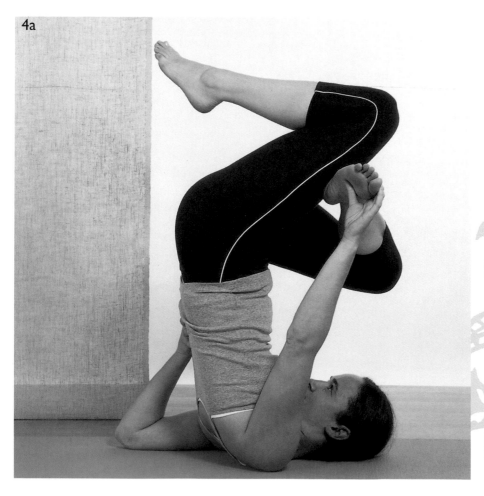

## 4 High Lotus Pose

*Urdhva Padmasana*

**Inhale:** straighten your knees and lift both legs back into the All Limbs Pose (see p. 104).

**Exhale:** bend your right leg and place your right ankle on top of your left thigh (see 4a), then bend your left leg and pull the foot on top of your right thigh, into

4b

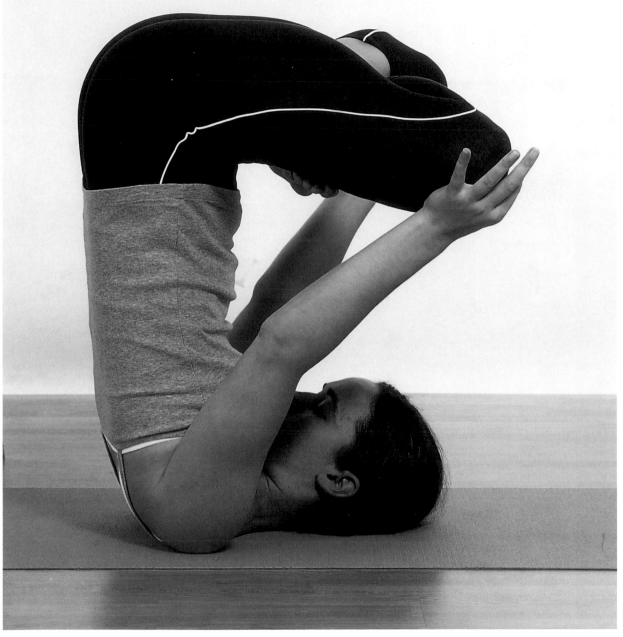

the Lotus Pose (see p. 115). Your knees and thighs should be parallel to the floor. Hold your knees with both hands and straighten your arms (see 4b). Apply both bandhas.

**Breath:** hold for 10 breaths.

**Beginners:** if it is not possible to get into the Lotus Pose, bend your knees and lightly cross your legs.

**BENEFITS:** this pose purifies the colon and urinary tract, while the anterior part of the spinal column becomes strong.

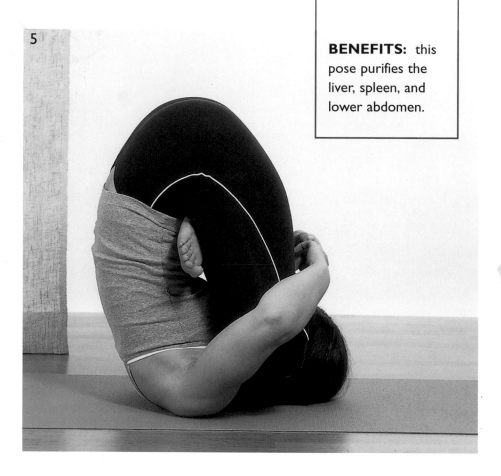

5

BENEFITS: this pose purifies the liver, spleen, and lower abdomen.

## 5 Embryo Pose
*Pindasana*

**Exhale:** bring both knees toward your head. Put both arms around your legs and draw them in as close as possible to your body, catching hold of your left wrist with your right hand.
**Breath:** remain in this position for 10 breaths.

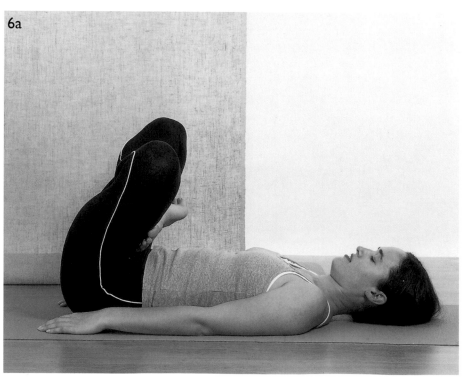

6a

## 6 Fish Pose
*Matsyasana*

**Inhale:** release your legs and place your arms on the floor away from your body, with both palms facing down. Very slowly, one vertebra at a time, roll your body back down to the floor, without lifting your head, until your entire back is flat on the floor, with your legs still in the Lotus Pose (see 6a). Then lift yourself up onto your elbows, lower

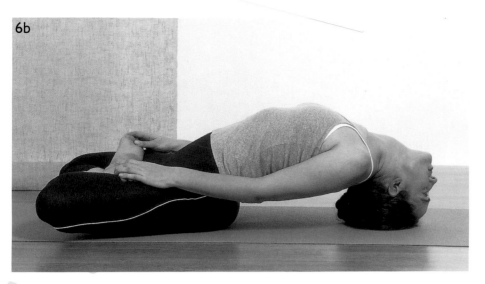

6b

**BENEFITS:** both this pose and the following one act as a counterpose to the All Limbs cycle and remove any kinks in the neck (plus potential shoulder or waist pain) as a result of the practice of this cycle. Both poses also purify the liver, esophagus, and spleen.

your knees to the floor and at the same time raise your head, arching your back and placing the crown of your head on the floor. Lift your chest, straighten your arms, and take hold of your feet (see 6b).

**Breath:** remain in this position for 10 breaths.

## 7 Extended Foot Pose *Uttana Padasana*

**Exhale:** release your feet and legs and lie flat on the floor.
**Inhale:** lift both feet off the floor at an angle of 45°, with your toes pointing away from your head. Bring the palms of your hands together and lift both arms so that they are parallel to your legs. Keep your chest raised and the crown of your head on the floor.

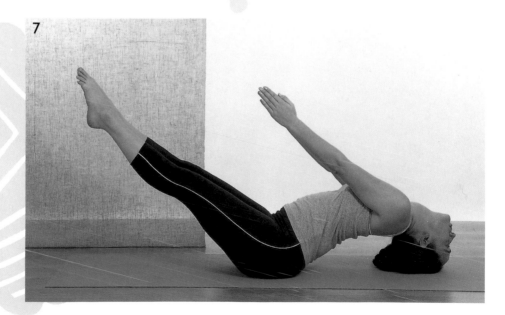

7

Keep all the muscles in your body taught.
**Breath:** remain in this position for 10 breaths.
**Inhale:** release the pose and lie flat on the floor.

**Exhale:** lift your legs into the Plow Pose (see p. 105), placing your hands palms down on the floor on either side of your head. Roll backward into the Four-Limbed

Stick (see p. 38) for a Half-Vinyasa (see p. 72).
**Beginners:** you can sit up and perform a Half-Vinyasa without having to roll backward.

# fast index to the All Limbs cycle

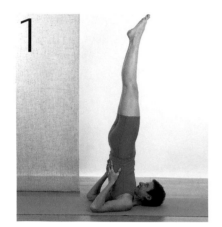

**1**

All Limbs Pose

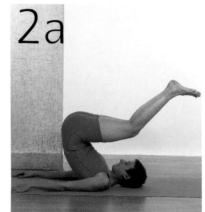

**2a**

Plow Pose

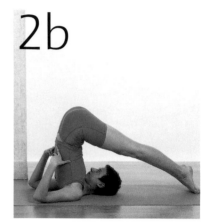

**2b**

Plow Pose

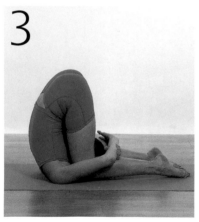

**3**

Ear-Pressure Pose

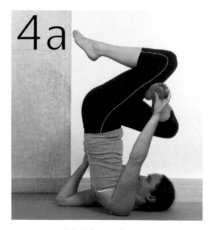

**4a**

High Lotus Pose

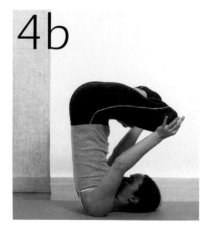

**4b**

High Lotus Pose

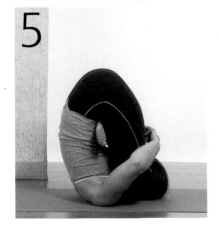

**5**

Embryo Pose

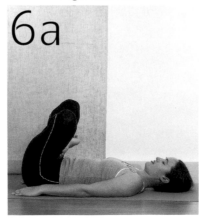

**6a**

Fish Pose

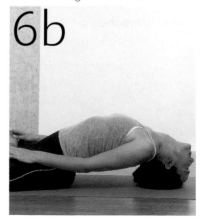

**6b**

Fish Pose

7

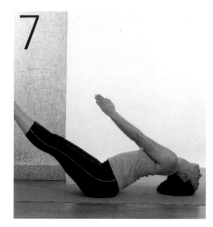

Extended Foot Pose

**BENEFITS:** the All Limbs pose brings a fresh supply of blood to all the essential organs of the body, revitalizing the entire system. It particularly stimulates the thyroid and parathyroid glands, which are situated in the neck and regulate the hormones, so this pose brings balance to both body and mind. It relieves asthma, congestion, and breathing-related problems, soothes the entire nervous system, and relieves hypertension, irritation, insomnia, and headaches.

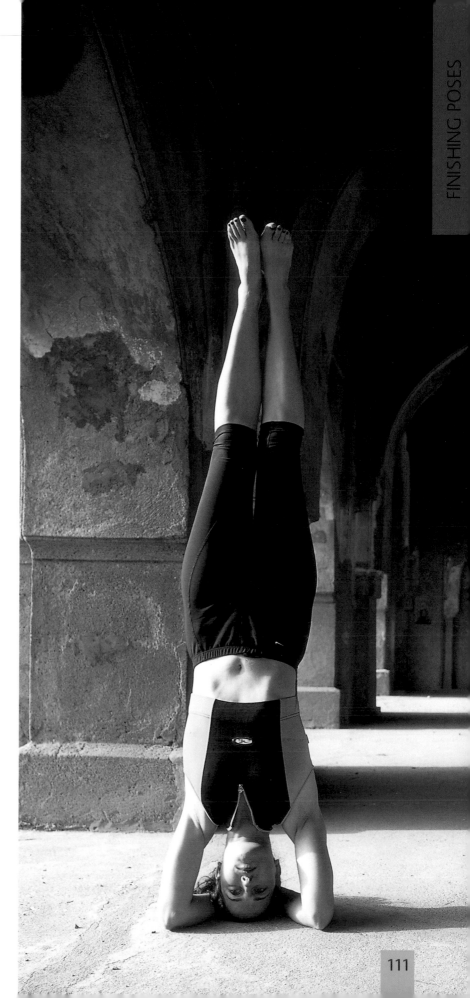

111

# The Headstand cycle

*The headstand is referred to as as the "king" of all asanas. The head contains the brain, which controls the nervous system and is the seat of the mind. Just as a country can prosper only under the guidance of a wise ruler, so the health of the body is dependent on the health of the mind.*

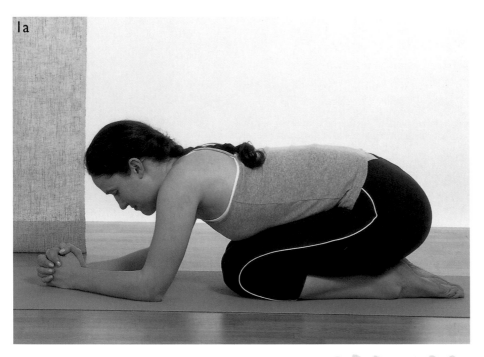

1a

**Beginners:** bend your knees to your chest once your torso is vertical, then find your balance and straighten your legs.
**Breath:** keep your breathing even and regular, and on no account hold your breath. With practice this pose can be held for up to three hours. However, beginners should remain for just 25 breaths. Advanced practitioners should remain in this pose for at least five minutes to obtain the maximum benefits.
**Inhale:** lift your head and put the entire weight of your body onto your forearms.
**Exhale:** release your head to the floor and slowly lower your feet back down.

**Headstand Pose**
*Salamba Sirasana*
**Inhale:** jump from the Half-Vinyasa (see p. 72) to a kneeling position. Rest your forearms on the floor with your elbows the same distance apart as your shoulders. Interlock your fingers (see 1a).

**Exhale:** place the crown of your head on the floor so that your palms touch the back of your head. Straighten your legs and walk your feet in toward your head until your torso is vertical. Tighten your knees, then lift both legs off the floor with the strength of your abdominal muscles and by pressing your forearms into the floor (see 1b). Tighten the leg and torso muscles and point your toes (see 1c). Apply mula and uddiyana bandha (see p. 25).

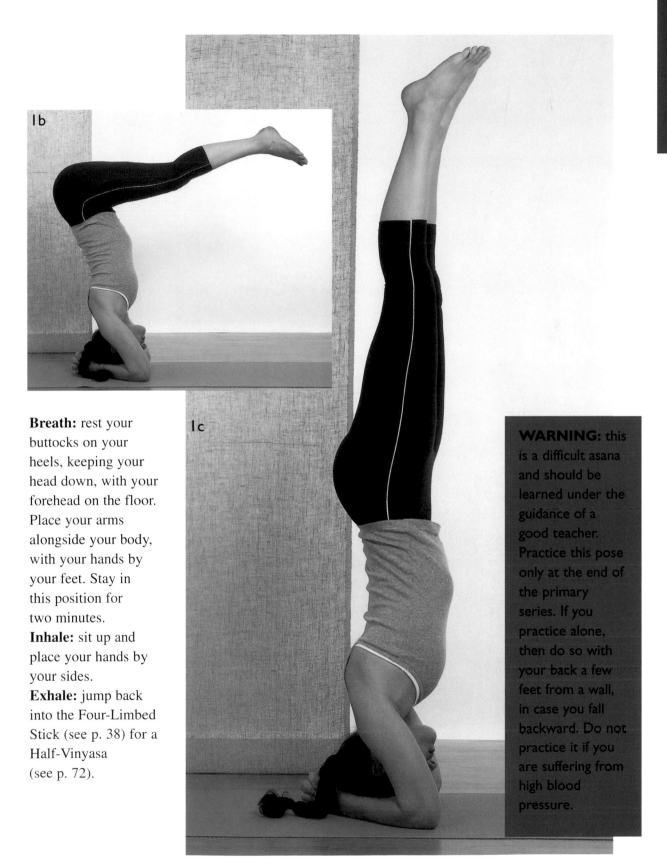

1b

1c

**Breath:** rest your buttocks on your heels, keeping your head down, with your forehead on the floor. Place your arms alongside your body, with your hands by your feet. Stay in this position for two minutes.

**Inhale:** sit up and place your hands by your sides.

**Exhale:** jump back into the Four-Limbed Stick (see p. 38) for a Half-Vinyasa (see p. 72).

**WARNING:** this is a difficult asana and should be learned under the guidance of a good teacher. Practice this pose only at the end of the primary series. If you practice alone, then do so with your back a few feet from a wall, in case you fall backward. Do not practice it if you are suffering from high blood pressure.

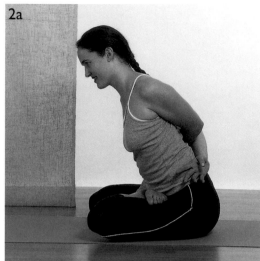

2a

## 2 Bound Lotus Pose

*Baddha Padmasana*

**Inhale:** jump into a sitting position.

**Exhale:** bend your right leg and place your right foot on top of your left thigh. Then bend your left leg and place your left foot on top of your right thigh. Bend forward and swing your left arm around your back, grabbing your left big toe (see 2a). Swing your right arm back, over the left, to grab your right big toe (see 2b).

**Inhale:** lift your chest, straighten your spine, and bend your head until your chin rests on your chest.

**Breath:** hold for 10 breaths.

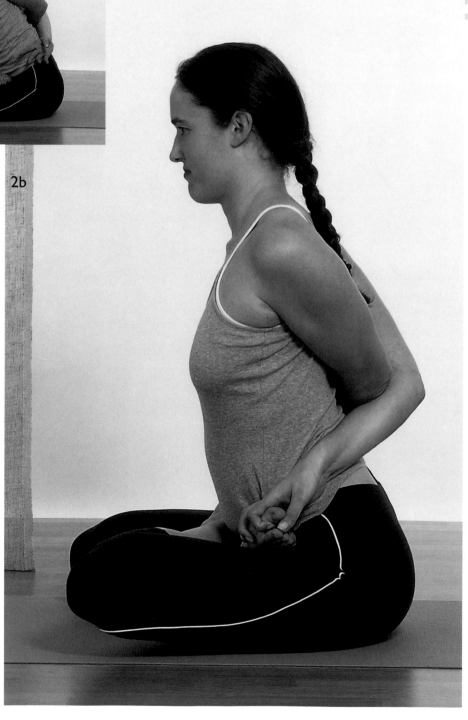

2b

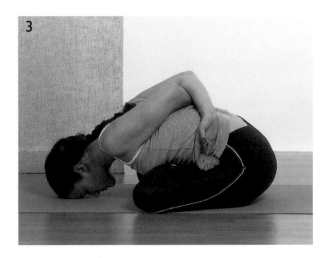

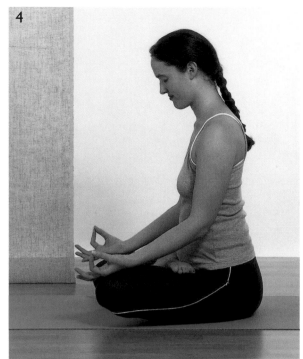

## 3 Yogic Seal
*Yoga Mudra*

**Exhale:** still holding your toes, bend as far forward as possible until your forehead (and eventually, with practice, your chin) rests on the floor.

**Breath:** hold this position for 10 breaths.

**Inhale:** lift your head and torso and release your toes.

**Exhale:** place both hands, palms down, about 12 inches/ 30 cm from your buttocks, with your fingers facing forward. Lift your chest and bend your head backward.

**Inhale:** come back to the center.

## 4 Lotus Pose
*Padmasana*

**Exhale:** place your hands on your knees, with your index fingers and thumbs touching and the backs of your hands resting on your knees. Tuck your chin in and bend your head slightly forward.

**Breath:** remain thus, focusing on your breathing for 25 breaths.

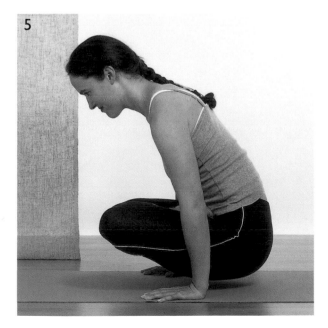

## 5 Upsprung Pose
*Utpluthih*

**Inhale:** place your hands, palms down, next to your buttocks and lift your torso and legs, still in the Lotus Pose, off the floor.

**Breath:** hold for 25 deep breaths.

**Exhale:** swing your legs back for a Half-Vinyasa (see p. 72). Finish with the Relax Pose (Savasana) (see p. 31).

# fast index to the Headstand cycle

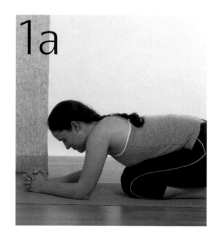

Headstand Pose

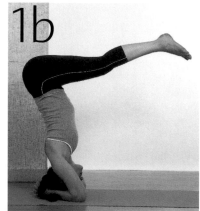

Headstand Pose

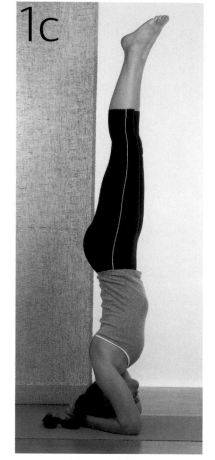

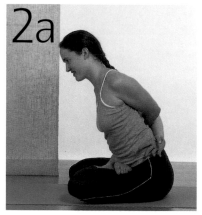

Bound Lotus Pose

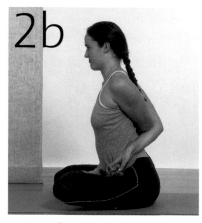

Bound Lotus Pose

Headstand Pose

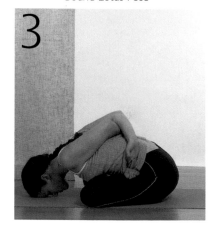

Yogic Seal

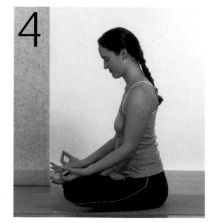

Lotus Pose

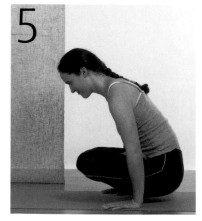

Upsprung Pose

# THE SUBTLE ENERGIES OF MUDRAS

*"In order, therefore, to awaken the goddess, who is sleeping at the entrance to Brahma's door, mudras should be practiced well."* Hatha Yoga Pradipika, ch. 3, v. 5

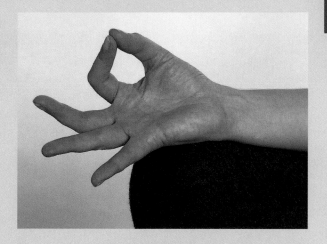

■ During yoga practice certain hand positions – referred to as mudras – are often adopted. The word mudra can be translated as "seal," meaning knowledge. Mudras are subtle physical movements that increase awareness and concentration. There are many different types of mudra in the yogic scriptures, some of which involve the whole body, while others are simple hand gestures. Generally mudras are said to manipulate prana, or energy flow, in the body. Hand mudras are meditation tools, which redirect the energy emitted through the hands back into the body.

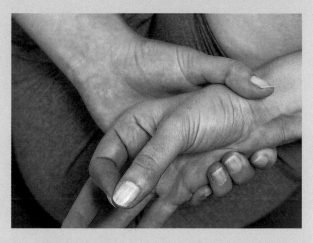

■ The Chin Mudra is a classic yogic meditation posture and is the gesture of consciousness. The palms of the hands face upwards while resting on the knees, and the tips of the thumbs and index fingers touch, while the remaining fingers are relaxed and slightly apart. The thumb- and finger-tips contain many nerve endings, and when they touch they create a circuit that sends energy back into the body. A variation of this is the Jnana Mudra, which is the gesture of knowledge. It has the same finger position, but the palms point downward rather than upward.

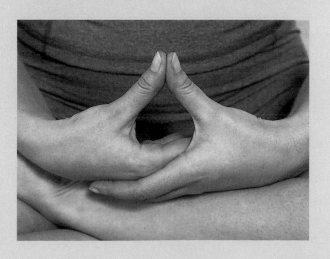

■ Bhairava Mudra, meaning "fierce gesture," is another mudra that you can assume during meditation. Sit in a comfortable cross-legged position and place your right palm on top of your left palm with the thumbs touching. Both hands then rest in your lap. The two hands represent the ida and pingala nadis (see p. 26), symbolizing the union of the individual with higher awareness.

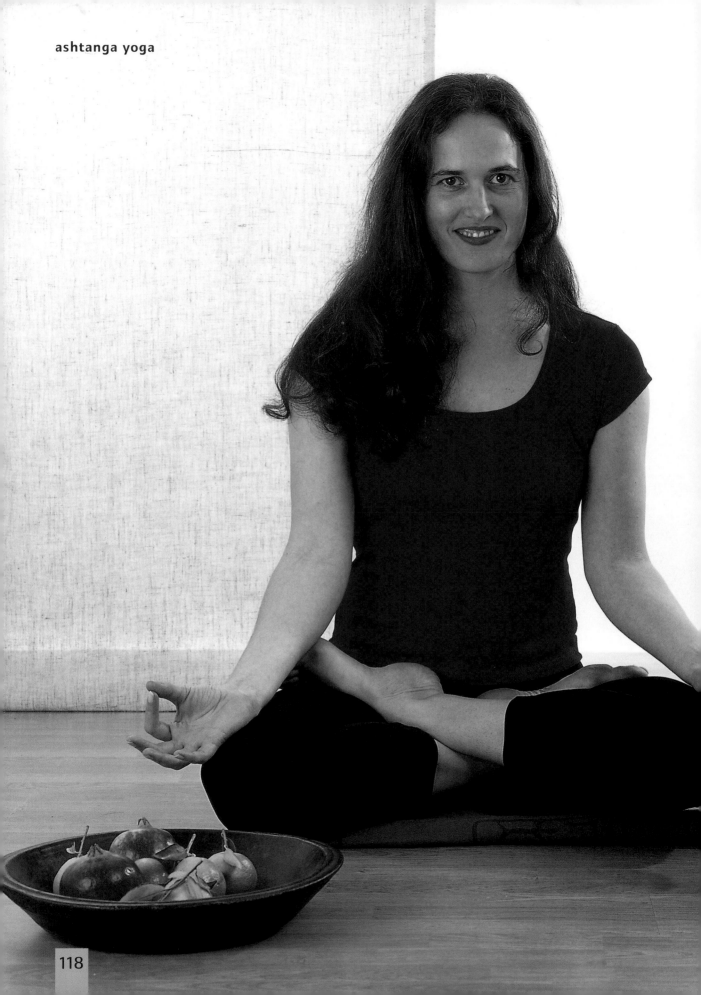

# CHAPTER FIVE

# Daily practice

The more energy and effort you put into your practice of yoga, the more you will benefit. Ashtanga yoga is a system of self-practice, and once you have learned the sequence from a qualified teacher, you then need to incorporate it into your daily schedule.

# Schedules

*Guruji's golden rule is to practice every day at the same time. There is a great advantage in doing this, in that you establish a rhythm and both prepare and focus the mind.*

Unfortunately most people do not have the luxury of being able to devote a great deal of time to yoga practice; instead, they have to fit it into an already busy schedule. However, you should commit yourself to practicing yoga at least two or three times a week.

The Ashtanga primary series takes time and patience to master. It is impossible to give a definite timescale in which to accomplish all the postures. Every individual holds tension in a different area of their body, and so different postures are either difficult or easy, depending on which areas of the body are tight. One person's medicine is often another's poison. Each individual has to work through their own weak points under the guidance of a teacher, but the postures must be practiced in sequence. Otherwise you do run the risk of disrupting the alignment of your body by strengthening certain muscles at the expense of others.

■ This section offers a weekly guide for beginners. The timetable provides a basic structure, but your teacher will advise you on your specific goals. If you come to a pose that you cannot do, do not force your body into it; that is your limit. Continue to practice all the preceding poses and keep including the difficult pose until you have mastered it.

■ With a little effort, most beginners can quite quickly get as far as Marici Pose A, at which point a plateau is often reached and progress seems minimal. Nevertheless, with regular practice of the postures, you will develop stamina and flexibility, preparing you for the more difficult part of the series: Sleeping Tortoise, Embryo in the Womb, Rooster Pose, and Bound Angle Pose (see pp. 82–85). After achieving these, the rest of the series should flow more easily until the back-bending sequence of the Bridge Pose and Upward Bow (see pp. 92–95). These poses are initially challenging, but they are important as they bend the spine backward and act as a counterbalance to all the forward bending of the primary series.

# WEEK ONE

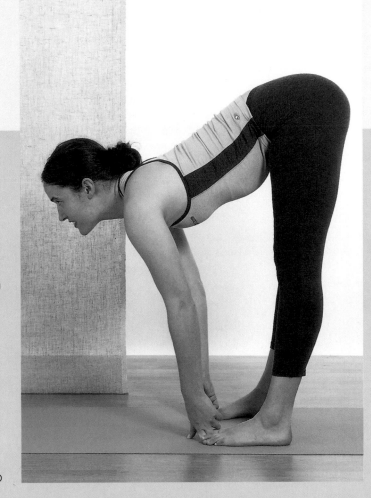

| | |
|---|---|
| **Days 1–3** | Begin by practicing Salute to the Sun A and B (see pp. 36–51). These two series form an excellent warm-up sequence. It is important to focus on breathing in rhythm with the series of poses, to create a natural flow. These asanas can be practiced on their own to get a feel for Ashtanga yoga before seeking a teacher, but if you are an absolute beginner you should then find a teacher to guide you through the rest of the series. Always end your practice with the Relax Pose (see p. 31). |
| **Day 4** | After the warm-up sequence, begin working on the Forward Bends (see pp. 54–55). These two poses help to open and elongate the hamstrings at the backs of the legs. End your practice with the Relax Pose. |
| **Day 5** | Add the Extended Triangle (see p. 56) to your series. This opens and stretches the sides of the body. End your practice with the Relax Pose. |
| **Day 6** | By the sixth day you should be beginning to feel the benefits of the forward and sideways stretches and have more mobility in your upper body. Add the Reversed Triangle (see p. 56), which is a spinal twist, giving more flexibility to your spine. For beginners the most difficult aspect of this pose is balance and you will need a teacher or partner present to hold you steady. If you want to practice this asana on your own, then do so against a wall for balance. End your practice with the Relax Pose. |

# WEEK TWO

■ This week adds more standing poses to complete the basics of the primary series. It also introduces some standing balances, as well as recapping on what you have learned so far.

| | |
|---|---|
| **Day 1** | Practice all the exercises recommended so far and add the Extended Sideways Pose (see p. 57). This stretches both sides of the body. Finish with the Relax Pose (see p. 31). |
| **Day 2** | Add the four variations of the Spread-Leg Pose (see pp. 57–59). These asanas really help to stretch the backs and insides of the legs and extend the spine. End your practice with the Relax Pose. |
| **Day 3** | If you are able to do all the poses so far, then add the Sideways Extension (see p. 59). The standing positions up to now have built the foundation of the primary series. They tone and strengthen the legs and lower back and develop flexibility in the spine. Once these standing poses have been mastered, then you can practice the standing balances of the Thumb-to-Foot Pose (see p. 60) and the Half-Bound Lotus Stretch (see p. 62). End your practice with the Relax Pose. |
| **Days 4–6** | Practice all the standing poses that have been included so far. |

# WEEK THREE

■ This week perfects the standing balances and completes the standing poses, before going on to introduce the Half-Vinyasa – which will be used repeatedly from now on – and the first of the sitting poses.

| | |
|---|---|
| **Day 1** | Practice the standing poses and the Thumb-to-Foot Pose (see p. 60). Your teacher will assist you in this asana by holding your raised leg, but in time you will get your balance. If you want to practice the pose at home, you can use a window ledge to support your foot. End your practice with the Relax Pose (see p. 31). |
| **Day 2** | Add the Half-Bound Lotus Stretch (see p. 62). The full pose is a very difficult to master and, unless you are naturally flexible, requires time and effort. Initially you will need a |

# WEEK FOUR

■ If you have experienced no major obstacles thus far, then you can introduce more complex sitting poses. At this point your teacher may also acquaint you with the finishing poses, especially the All Limbs Pose.

| Day 1 | Practice all the postures learned so far and add the Half-Bound Foot (see p. 74). Again this is an awkward and difficult pose for beginners. It takes a while before your hip joints and knees open fully, but this pose prepares the body for the full Lotus Position and is a good pose for beginners to practice. Finish with the Relax Pose (see p. 31). |
|---|---|
| Day 2 | Add the Three-Limbed Forward Bend (see p. 75), which stretches and opens the lower back. End your practice with the Relax Pose. |
| Day 3 | Practice the poses learned so far. End your practice with the Relax Pose. |
| Day 4 | Introduce the Head-to-Knee poses (see pp. 76–77) under the guidance of your teacher. End your practice with the Relax Pose. |
| Day 5 | Begin by working on Head-to-Knee Pose C (see p. 77), which is another initially awkward pose but becomes much easier with practice. Add Marici Pose A (see p. 78), although it may take time before you are able to catch hold of your hand behind your back. End your practice with the Relax Pose. |
| Day 6 | Practice all that you have learned so far. End your practice with the Relax Pose. |

| | teacher to assist you in holding the foot and in balancing while bending forward. End your practice with the Relax Pose. |
|---|---|
| Day 3 | Practice all the poses that you have learned so far. End your practice with the Relax Pose. |
| Day 4 | Add the Uneven Pose (see p. 63) and the Warrior Pose sequence (see pp. 64–65). Together these make up a fluid series of movements and complete the standing series. End your practice with the Relax Pose. |
| Day 5 | Do all the standing postures learned so far, then try jumping through to a sitting position, the Half-Vinyasa (see p. 72). Add the Back Extension (see p. 73) and the counterpose Forward Extension (see p. 74). End your practice with the Relax Pose. |
| Day 6 | Practice everything you have learned so far. End your practice with the Relax Pose. |

# Spiritual changes

*Yoga is the science of mind and body. Initially we may practice yoga physically and understand it intellectually, but it will only become true knowledge once it is "realized" – that is, experienced through a deeper internal understanding.*

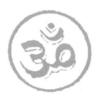  

Spirituality is actually a form of knowledge. There are many levels of understanding, known as bhumis, in the yoga scriptures. Through realization, yoga becomes integrated into all our actions. It is not enough to practice yoga for an hour in the morning, feel relaxed, then find yourself getting angry and upset later in the day. Yoga provides the tools to enable you to change your attitudes. No situation is entirely positive or negative, but is colored by your perceptions, which you have the ability to alter. The increased awareness that yoga develops should be applied to all aspects of life. Then it becomes wisdom: a means of inner guidance.

## ABANDONING THE FRUITS OF OUR ACTIONS

Usually our minds are fragmented, filled with thoughts of future activities or past events. Yoga teaches us to bring our awareness to the present moment, to be fully involved in whatever we undertake, without thought of the final goal. The fruits of our actions are offered instead to the divine spirit.

## GAINING EQUANIMITY

By practicing the asanas and working with our breathing through the most difficult postures, equanimity emerges. In our daily affairs we are then able to remain neutral or balanced through the dualities of gain and loss, victory and defeat, fame and shame. We are no longer tossed about by the vicissitudes of life.

## SERVICE TO OTHERS

When we discovers our inner source of strength and clarity, we become internally free. Recognizing the divine spark within ourself, we have complete self-reliance. Then we have a practical knowledge that can be of benefit to others.

Regardless of whether or not you are seeking spiritual knowledge, yogic practices can give tangible results. Yoga develops physical health and mental

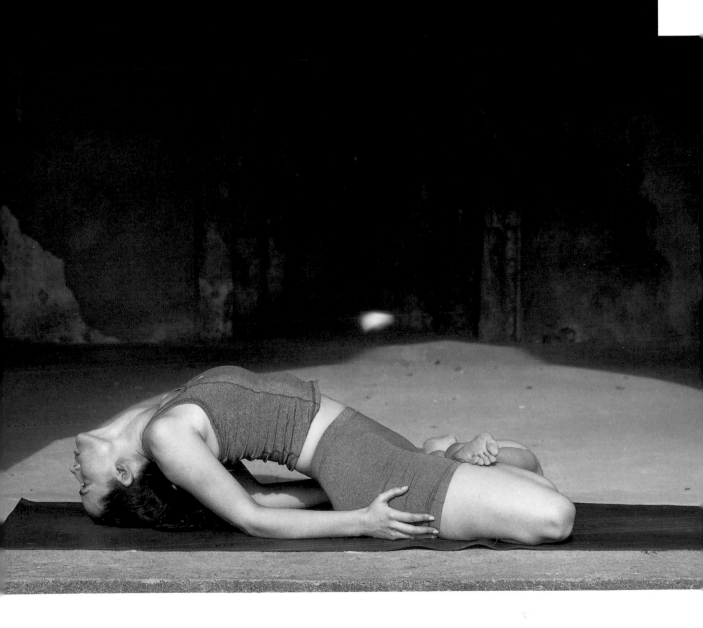

equilibrium in an increasingly stressful society. With increased awareness, life begins to flow smoothly from one event to the next without unnecessary anxiety. Asana practice helps to remove the strain that accumulates from doing a desk job. If practiced properly, yoga detoxifies the body, bringing new vital energy, which rejuvenates the whole system. Yoga draws the body, mind, and spirit into greater harmony, providing a deep sense of contentment and wellbeing.

# Glossary

| | |
|---|---|
| *agni* | Internal fire. |
| *asana* | A yoga pose or posture; the asanas form the third "limb" of Ashtanga yoga. |
| *Ashtanga yoga* | A form of yoga founded by Guru Shri Pattabhi Jois, meaning eight steps or "limbs." |
| *atman* | The transcendental soul, from the Sanskrit word for "breath." |
| *bandha* | An internal "lock" or muscular contraction that helps the practice of yoga. |
| *chakra* | One of seven energy centres or "wheels" lying along the sushumna nadi. |
| *dharana* | Concentration, forming the sixth "limb" of Ashtanga yoga. |
| *dhyana* | Meditation or a deepening of concentration, the seventh "limb" of Ashtanga yoga. |
| *drishti* | A steady gaze – fixing your gaze on a single point, without distraction, forms part of the sixth "limb" of Ashtanga yoga. |
| *Gheranda Samhita* | One of the foremost ancient texts on yoga. |
| *granthi* | A psychic knot. |
| *guru* | A teacher or leader who gives spiritual guidance to his disciples. |
| *Half-Vinyasa* | A series of movements used between the sitting poses in Ashtanga yoga. |
| *Hatha yoga* | A classic school of yoga, meaning forceful or physical yoga, comprising the asanas. |
| *Hatha Yoga Pradipika* | A foremost ancient text on Hatha yoga, written by the yogi Swatmarama. |
| *ida nadi* | A nadi associated with mental faculties and female energy. |
| *Guru Shri Pattabhi Jois (Guruji)* | The founder of Ashtanga yoga. |
| *khanda* | The foundation of the body, at the base of the spine, where the kundalini energy is stored. |
| *Krishna-macharya* | A 20th-century yogi and philosopher who inspired renewed interest in yoga throughout India. |
| *kundalini* | The cosmic energy that lies dormant in each person. |
| *Laya yoga* | Visualization or forming a mental image – used to aid physical relaxation. |
| *mantra* | A sacred word or phrase, such as "OM," used to focus the mind. |
| *mudra* | A hand position or subtle physical movement that increases awareness and concentration. |
| *mula bandha* | The root lock, one of the most important internal locks. |
| *nadi* | One of at least 72,000 subtle energy channels that run throughout the body. |
| *niyamas* | The "devotions" or observances that form the second "limb" of Ashtanga yoga. |
| *Patanjali* | The Indian sage who founded the yoga system, compiled in the four books of his *Yoga Sutra*. |
| *pingala nadi* | A nadi associated with physical faculties and masculine energy. |
| *prana* | Life force – a subtle energy that pervades all phenomena and flows throughout the subtle body via the nadis. |
| *pranayama* | Breath control, or breathing exercises that cleanse and strengthen |

| | |
|---|---|
| | the mind and body; it forms the fourth "limb" of Ashtanga yoga. |
| *pratyahara* | Withdrawal of the senses, which forms the fifth "limb" of Ashtanga yoga. |
| *Puranas* | Ancient Sanskrit chronicles, possibly dating as far back as 6000 B.C. |
| *Raja yoga* | The "royal" path of yoga, or mind control, comprising the inner practices of the eight steps or "limbs" of Ashtanga yoga. |
| *Relax Pose* | The pose lying on the flat of the back in which each asana practice should finish, to relax and rebalance the body. |
| *Vamana Rishi* | An Indian sage who transcribed an intricate system of linked yoga poses, possibly more than 2,000 years ago. |
| *sadhana* | Spiritual practice, or a means of self-realization. |
| *samadhi* | Enlightenment or self-realization the eighth "limb" of Ashtanga yoga and the ultimate goal. |
| *shakti-pata* | Direct spiritual transmission of knowledge from one generation to the next. |
| *Shiva* | A popular Hindu deity referred to in the *Puranas* as the founder of yoga; Shiva is one of the three chief deities, and the god of personal destiny. |
| *sloka* | A verse. |
| *sushumna nadi* | The most important nadi, which runs along the body's central channel or spinal column. |
| *tattvas* | The five elements of fire, water, earth, air, and ether, which can be observed during Ashtanga practice. The earth element is the asana, or the various poses. Fire is the internal heat that is produced. Water appears as the sweat, and air as the ujjui breathing. Ether is the concentration necessary for the practice. |
| *third eye* | The ajna-chakra, situated in the center of the head between the eyebrows; it often forms a point of focus in Ashtanga yoga. |
| *uddiyana banda* | The "flying contraction," one of the most important internal locks or bandhas. |
| *ujjayi breathing* | A system of breath control taught by Guruji that forms a vital integral part of Ashtanga yoga; literally "victorious breath." |
| *vinyasa* | Breath-synchronized movement. |
| *yamas* | The restraints that form the first "limb" of Ashtanga yoga, consisting of five abstentions. |
| *yoga chikitsa* | Literally, "yoga therapy" – the primary or beginners' series in the Ashtanga system. |
| *Yoga Korunta* | An ancient Sanskrit text written by Vamana Rishi. |
| *Yoga Sutra* | The four books written by Patanjali that provide the blueprint for the eight steps of Ashtanga yoga. |
| *yogi* | A male master of yoga. |
| *yogini* | A female master of yoga. |

# Index